The Pocket Guide to Dog Tricks

The Pocket Guide to Dog Tricks

Kyra Sundance

QUARRY

© 2018 Quarto Publishing Group USA Inc.
Text © 2007, 2009, 2010, 2011, 2014, 2017, 2018 Kyra Sundance

First Published in 2018 by Quarry Books, an imprint of The Quarto Group,
100 Cummings Center, Suite 265-D, Beverly, MA 01915, USA.
T (978) 282-9590 F (978) 283-2742 QuartoKnows.com

Quarry Books titles are also available at discount for retail, wholesale, promotional, and bulk
purchase. For details, contact the Special Sales Manager by email at specialsales@quarto.
com or by mail at The Quarto Group, Attn: Special Sales Manager, 401 Second Avenue North,
Suite 310, Minneapolis, MN 55401, USA.

10 9 8 7 6 5 4 3 2 1

ISBN: 978-1-63159-569-1

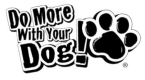

Digital edition published in 2018

The content in this book previously appeared in the following titles published by Quarry Books:
101 Dog Tricks (2007), *51 Puppy Tricks* (2009), *101 Ways to Do More with Your Dog* (2010),
10-Minute Dog Training Games (2011), *101 Dog Tricks, Kids Edition* (2014), and *Dog Training
101* (2017).

Library of Congress Cataloging-in-Publication Data available

Design/Page Layout: Kyra Sundance
Photography: Slickforce Studios

Printed in China

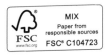

MIX
Paper from
responsible sources
FSC® C104723

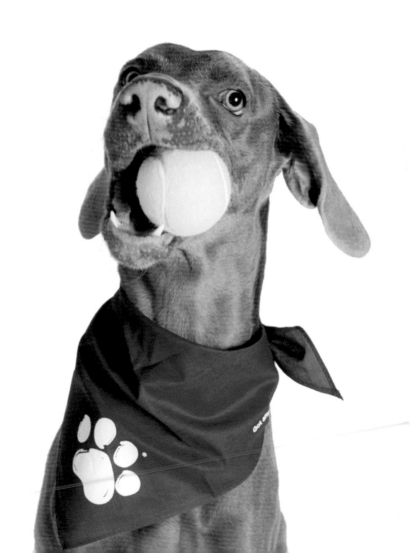

CONTENTS

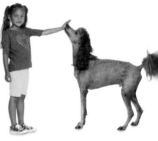

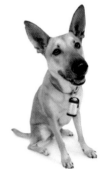

PAWS UP

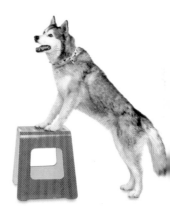

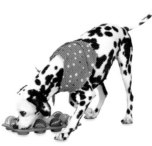

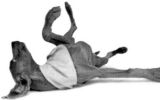

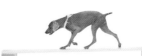

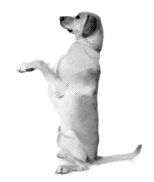

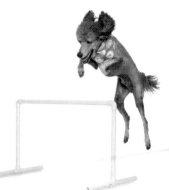

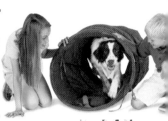

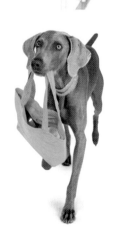

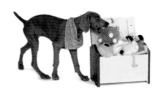

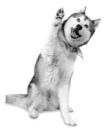

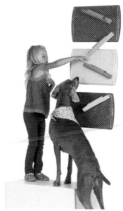

AUTHOR'S NOTE

A dog family member can enrich our lives in so many ways: by giving us companionship and love, by engaging us in lighthearted play, and by spreading joy and enthusiasm.

With this book you will use positive training methods to build a joyful relationship with your dog, where he is a willing partner in the training process. Training builds relationships by deepening communication pathways, trust, and mutual respect. It offers a way to bond with your dog as you strive toward common goals. The trust and cooperative spirit developed through this process will last a lifetime.

I hope this book helps to enhance your relationship with your dog and encourages you to "Do More With Your Dog!®"

Kyra Sundance

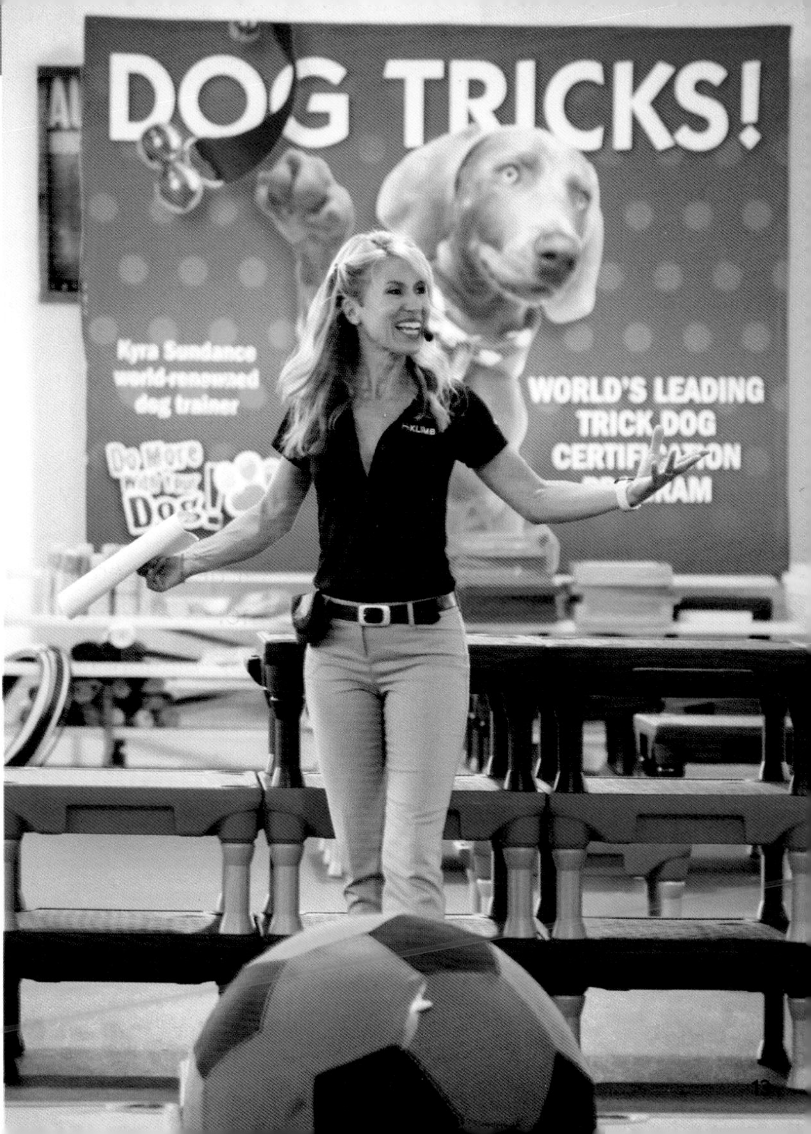
DOG TRICKS!
Kyra Sundance
world-renowned
dog trainer
WORLD'S LEADING
TRICK DOG

HOW TO USE THIS BOOK

This pocket guide contains 101 dog tricks organized by similarity. Teach the first trick in any chapter, and the other tricks in that chapter will build on that skill.

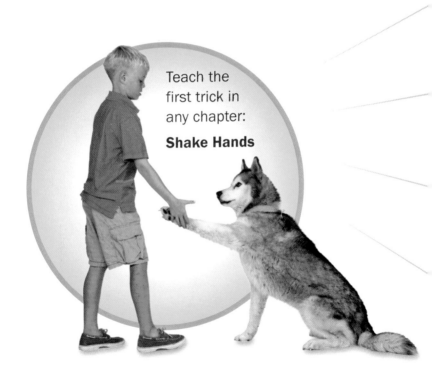

Teach the first trick in any chapter:

Shake Hands

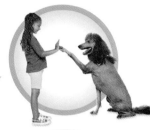

Once your dog can **shake hands**, rotate your palm vertically to teach him to **High-5**

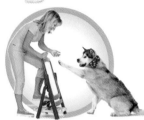

Pull your hand away at the last second to teach him **Pawprint Painting**

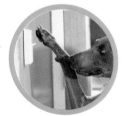

Have him shake hands at the wall to teach him to **Turn Off the Light**

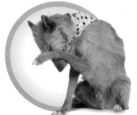

Shake hands on his muzzle to teach **Hide Your Eyes**

Trick training is about more than cute party tricks to entertain your friends. Trick training offers an opportunity to better understand how your dog thinks and have him better understand your cues. It deepens paths of communication, built through repetition and effort.

CAN ANY DOG LEARN TRICKS?

Sure! You'll find that the more tricks your dog knows, the quicker he'll pick up new ones. In a sense, you've taught him how to learn.

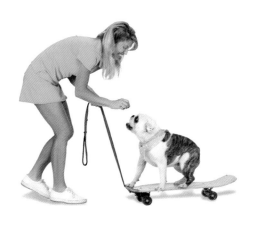

PUT IN THE TIME

When teaching a new trick, it often appears that your dog is not getting the concept and has no idea what the desired behavior is. He'll be squirming and pawing and obsessing over the treat in your hand. You might feel as if he will never understand. Don't stress it. Go through the same motions day after day, and one day you'll see a lightbulb go off in his head. That's the moment that truly bonds you with your dog.

HOW LONG DOES IT TAKE TO TRAIN A DOG?

How many years does it take for a child to become educated? For an athlete to become skilled? How many piano lessons until you're a musician? Dog training should be thought of as a lifelong process. Although at some point your dog will be able to produce a behavior on cue, he will still need repetition and refinement to maintain and improve his skills. Challenge your dog with new skills for the rest of his life, and you'll find your bond will increase tenfold.

BASIC TRAINING PRINCIPLES

POSITIVE TRAINING METHODS

In this book we use positive training methods which foster a happy, eager dog who strives to learn. Positive training techniques are not only humane and kind, but also are the fastest and easiest way to train a dog.

Provide a consistent and motivating environment for your dog as you guide him through each new trick. Reward each of his small successes along the way and use your "happy voice" to encourage and praise him.

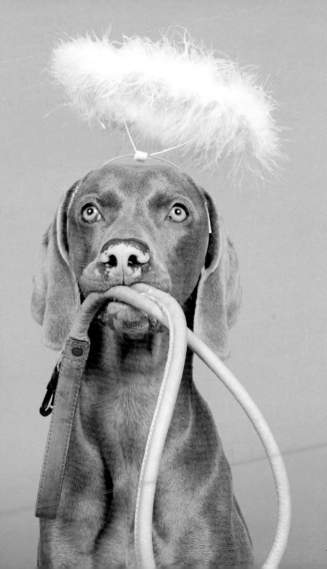

FOOD TREATS

Although a reward for a dog can be a toy, play, or praise, we usually use food treats because they are a high-value reward and can be dispensed quickly. During the learning stages of a new trick, you want to make it very rewarding for your dog by giving lots of treats for every small success. In fact, you may give your dog his entire dinner, piece by piece, during a ten-minute training session.

Keep your dog extra motivated by using "people food" treats, such as pea-size pieces of chicken, steak, cheese, goldfish crackers, noodles, or meatballs. Try microwaving hot dog slices on a paper-towel-covered plate for three minutes for a tasty treat!

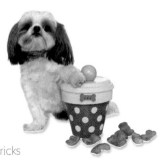

LURE, DON'T MANIPULATE

There are two obvious ways to get a dog into a desired position: you can lure him by encouraging him to follow a treat, or you can physically manipulate him into position. It is tempting to manipulate your dog's body physically; however, it can actually delay the learning process, as the dog is not required to engage his brain and is not learning the motor skills necessary to position his body himself. It is always preferable to lure your dog to position his body himself.

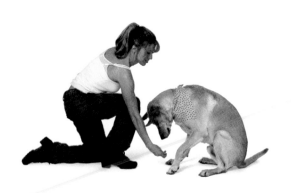

REWARD SUCCESS, IGNORE THE REST

One of the key skills your dog will develop through trick training is his ability to problem-solve through experimentation. Encourage your dog to try a lot of behaviors and let him know (with a treat) which ones were correct.

Trick training allows the dog to be silly and encourages independent action. You want to keep the enthusiasm high during training sessions or your dog could shut down for fear of being wrong. If your dog is giving you an incorrect behavior, it is probably not intentional. Instead of "no," try a more lighthearted "whoops!"

TIMING

During the learning process, your dog may squirm and try a variety of different things. You need to let him know immediately if each thing he tried was a success (treat) or nonsuccess (no treat). The key to helping him understand the goal behavior is to give him the treat at the exact moment that he performed correctly. Be ready with a treat in your hand and release it the instant your dog performs correctly. Don't reward five seconds after he has done the behavior, as your dog may not understand what he did to earn the reward.

MARKER TRAINING

It can sometimes be logistically difficult to reward your dog at the exact moment he performed correctly. But you *can* use a specific word (or a clicker) at that exact moment to let your dog know the instant he earned his reward. We call this special sound a **reward marker** because it marks the instant your dog earned a reward. A reward marker is always quickly followed by a treat. Some trainers use a reward marker of "good!" or "yes!"

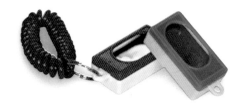

KEEP SESSIONS SHORT

Dogs have short attention spans. Don't train past the point where your dog has lost interest. Several five-minute sessions per day are ideal for most novice dogs.

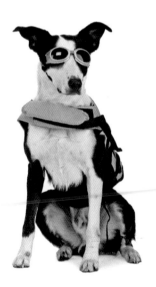

YOUR JOB AS A TRAINER

Your job as a trainer is to guide your dog in a consistent and motivating environment.

GUIDANCE

Guide your dog through the process of executing a new behavior, rewarding baby steps along the way. The goal of each training session is to get better results than the last time.

CONSISTENCY

Know the behavior you are looking for, and don't be wishy-washy. Use the same voice and intonation each time you give a verbal cue and enunciate clearly.

MOTIVATION

Think about an athletic coach. Is his job merely to plan the training schedule and tape it to the locker room door? No! He inspires, motivates, and encourages! He is upbeat when you are discouraged and slaps your shoulder with a "good job!" when you need it. You serve the same purpose for your dog. Every bit of enthusiasm you inject into your dog training will speed up his learning. And when your dog does something right use your high-pitched "happy voice" (yes, men, you have one too) to exude your delight!

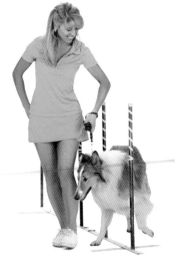

MOTIVATORS/REWARDS

"Shouldn't my dog want to learn tricks merely to please me?" Dogs do, in general, want to please their owners—but learning is hard!

A motivator, or reward, can come in different forms—a food morsel, favorite toy, or praise. In this book, the steps rely mostly on food treats. Food is enjoyed by all dogs, is quick to dispense and be swallowed, and is a clear way to signal a correct response. During the beginning stages of learning, a toy can be a distraction, as it takes a while for you to take it back and get your dog to regain focus. Praise is great, but can be arbitrary and unclear. Use a small but tasty food treat to reward the desired behavior.

DO I HAVE TO CARRY AROUND TREATS FOR THE REST OF MY LIFE?

Before worrying about emptying our pockets of treats, we need to make the behavior an automatic response. No matter how it is achieved, if you tell your dog to "sit" 500 times, and he sits, it becomes an automatic response. For the first 500 times, he was sitting because you were tempting him with a treat. Later, however, his muscle memory just hears the word "sit" and does it! It is at this point that you can start weaning your dog off his expectation of a reward. Rather than weaning completely off treats, however, use them as sporadic rewards.

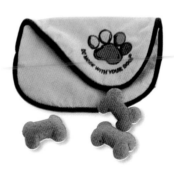

UPPING THE ANTE

The purpose of a treat is to reward a good effort. In kindergarten, a child gets a gold star for printing her name. In first grade, she only gets a gold star if she prints it neatly, and in second grade cursive is required for that same reward. What may have earned your dog a treat in the past, may no longer be enough to earn that treat today. We call this "upping the ante."

When first learning to shake a paw, reward your dog for barely lifting his paw, or for batting your hand. Once he has the hang of this, withhold the treat until he lifts his paw higher, or holds it longer. Every time your dog is achieving a step with about 75 percent success, up the ante and demand a higher skill to earn the treat.

HELP YOUR DOG BE SUCCESSFUL

The key to keeping your dog motivated is to keep him challenged, achieving regular successes. Try not to let your dog be wrong more than two or three times in a row, or he could become discouraged and not wish to perform. Instead, go back to an easier step for a while.

REGRESSION IS PART OF PROGRESSION

The key to keeping your dog motivated is to keep him challenged and achieving regular successes. If your dog goes for thirty seconds without getting a treat, he could become discouraged and not wish to continue. If your dog is struggling, temporarily lower the criteria for success. Regress back to an easier step where he can be successful for a while.

Your dog will go through spurts of learning and regression. Don't be reluctant to go back a step—it's usually only needed for a short while and will give your dog confidence to move forward.

GET IN THE RIGHT MINDSET

Dog training can be frustrating. Be prepared with your calm, patient attitude by reviewing these six rules:

RULE 1: BE FAIR

Treat your dog fairly by having rules that are specific, clear, and achievable—and consequences that are fair and predictable.

RULE 2: BE CONSISTENT

Be clear yourself about what you want; ask for it in a consistent way; and don't go back on your decisions.

RULE 3: MOTIVATE WITH POSITIVE REINFORCEMENT

Build a dog's motivation to please by rewarding his good behavior. Focus on solutions rather than problems. Help the dog develop a pattern of success and good behavior.

RULE 4: ATTENTION IS A REWARD

Recognize your attention toward your dog as the powerful reward that it is. Use it as a payoff for your dog's good behavior and withdraw it as a consequence for his inappropriate behavior.

RULE 5: DISCIPLINE

Discipline is not punishment and is not hurtful; it is the compassionate enforcement of fair rules. Discipline is a clear and consistent structure for you and your dog to understand expectations and consequences.

RULE 6: FORGIVE

Don't hold a grudge—deal with misbehavior and let it go. Always give your dog another chance to be a "good dog."

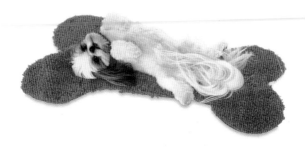

TOP 10 TRICK TRAINING TIPS

1. Reward with tasty treats
2. Reward while your dog is in the correct position
3. Reward immediately (no fishing in pockets)
4. Train before dinner
5. Train before playtime
6. End the session with your dog wanting more
7. Be consistent
8. Motivate—use your happy voice
9. Be patient—it won't happen overnight
10. Be a fun person to be around

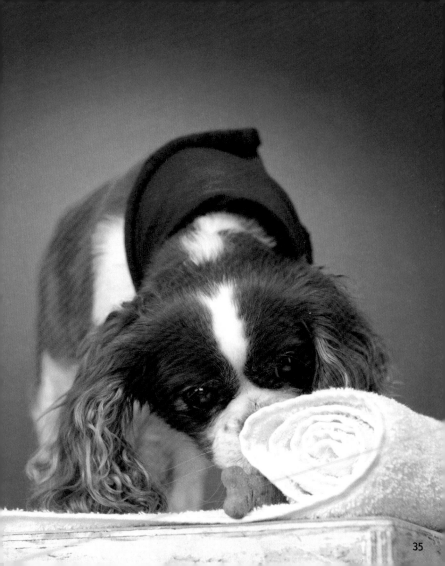

Touch My Hand

1. Wedge a treat between your fingers. Hold your hand flat, at your dog's nose height, with your palm toward your dog.

2. Say "touch!" and wiggle your hand to get your dog interested in the treat.

3. The second you feel his nose touch your hand, say "good!" and let him take the treat. Repeat this step a few times.

4. Once your dog gets the hang of this, try it with no treat between your fingers. Hold out your hand and say "touch!" The instant your dog touches your hand, say "good!" and give him a treat from your pocket.

TROUBLESHOOTING: Dogs love this game and catch on quickly. Avoid moving your hand toward your dog, but instead have him move his nose to you.

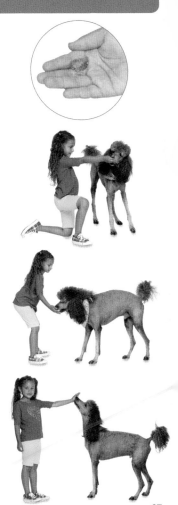

Touch a Target Stick

Teach your dog to touch a stick with his nose. This training tool can later be used to guide your dog into positions.

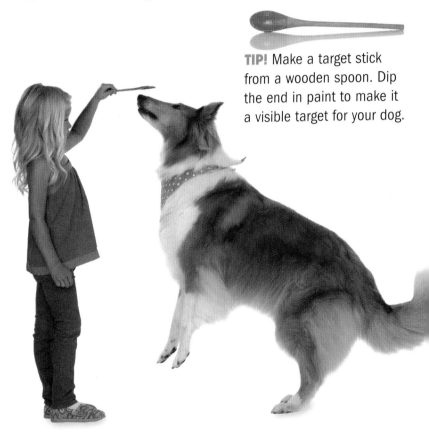

TIP! Make a target stick from a wooden spoon. Dip the end in paint to make it a visible target for your dog.

1. Put some treats in your pocket. Put a dab of peanut butter on the end of your target stick.

2. Hold out the stick to your dog. He will want to lick the peanut butter.

3. As soon as he touches the target stick, say "good!" and pull out a treat from your pocket.

4. After a few repetitions, try it without the peanut butter. The target stick will still smell like peanut butter, which should be enough to get your dog to sniff it. The instant he touches it, say "good!" and give him a treat.

WHAT TO EXPECT: Dogs learn this trick pretty quickly. Once your dog has the hang of it, hold the target stick at different heights, or have your dog follow a moving target.

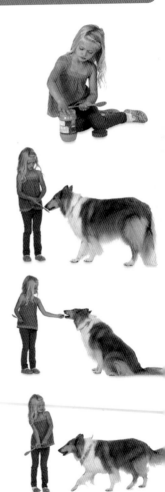

Close the Door

Teach your dog to push the door closed with his nose.

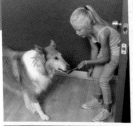

1. Have your dog **touch a target stick** (page 38) and give him a treat. Move the stick closer and closer to the door each time.

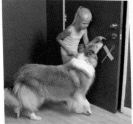

2. Tape the target stick to the door. Tap it or put a dab of peanut butter on it to encourage your dog to touch it. Don't forget to give a treat every time.

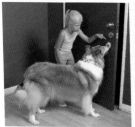

3. Replace the target stick with just a piece of colored tape. Use peanut butter on the tape if you need to.

4. Open the door slightly and ask your dog to "close the door." If he doesn't nose-touch the door hard enough to close it on the first try, encourage him to do it again. If he gets discouraged, go back to a previous step.

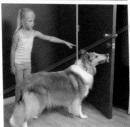

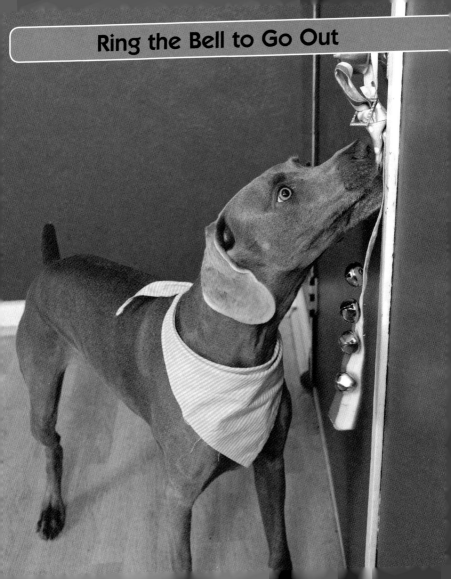

Ring the Bell to Go Out

1. Hang a bell from your doorknob and dab some peanut butter on it.

2. When your dog sniffs or licks it, it will jingle softly.

3. As soon as you hear the jingle, say "good!" and give her a treat.

4. Get your dog excited to go for a walk. Stop at the door and encourage her to ring the bell. It may take a while, but as soon as she touches the bell open the door and let her outside. Use the peanut butter again if you have to.

WHAT TO EXPECT: In the beginning, be very responsive to your dog's jingling and open the door every time she rings the bell. Dogs, even puppies, catch on quickly and learn to jingle the bell when they need to go out.

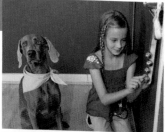

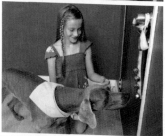

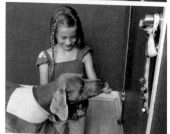

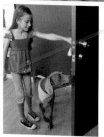

43

Roll Out the Carpet

Teach your dog to roll out the carpet. Hide treats inside the roll, and your dog will find a treat with every push.

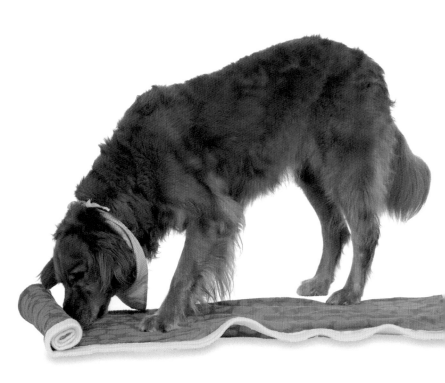

1. A hallway rug works great for this trick, but you can also use a blanket or a towel. Get a handful of strong smelling, small treats such as liver treats or pieces of beef jerky. Lay them in a line down the length of your rug.

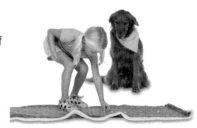

2. Roll up the rug with the treats inside.

3. Point out the first treat to your dog. As he nudges and unrolls the rug, it will reveal a treat. Each time he sniffs and nudges the rug, more treats will be revealed.

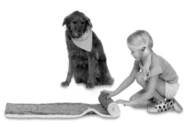

WHAT TO EXPECT: This is an easy game that any dog can learn. In the beginning, put lots of treats inside the rug, but as your dog gets better you can use treats, or even just one big treat at the end.

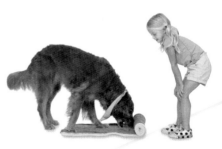

Soccer Ball Roll

Sports star dogs will get a kick out of this game, as they learn how to roll a soccer ball. Score!

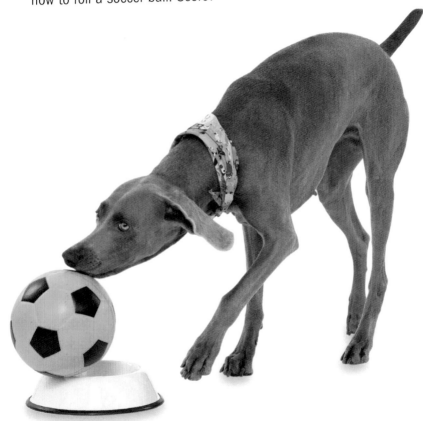

1. Show your dog as you drop a treat into her food bowl.

2. Place a soccer ball on top of the treat. Roll the ball off the treat a few times to make sure she knows the treat is still under there.

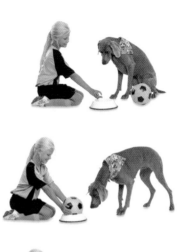

3. Give her a chance to figure out how to move the ball. She may use her nose or her paw.

4. When your dog finally gets the soccer ball out of the bowl, let her eat the treat as a reward.

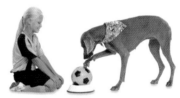

TROUBLESHOOTING: Some dogs don't like to be pushy. If your dog will not push the ball out of the bowl, try a lightweight inflatable ball instead, which will move with the slightest push from your dog.

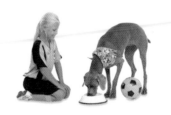

Treibball

Treibball is a competition sport in which a dog maneuvers a fitness ball into a goal. It originated as an activity that mimicked herding dogs prodding sheep into a pen.

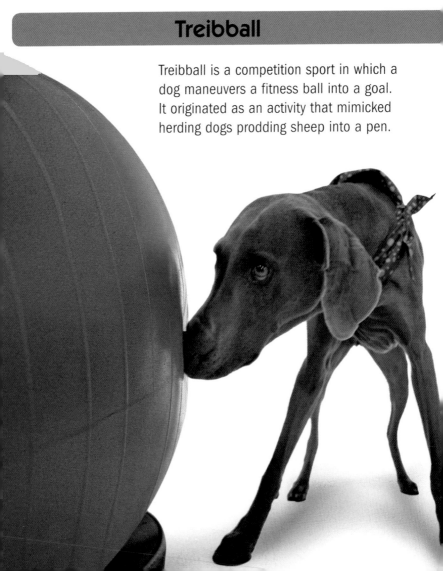

1. Construct a chute with two rails or by placing the back of a sofa parallel to a wall. Put the fitness ball at one end of the chute and place a treat at the base of the ball. As your dog reaches for the treat, she will bump the ball forward.

2. Drop additional treats in the chute behind the ball. Each time your dog bumps the ball, she will see the next treat.

3. Don't set any treats on the floor this time, but encourage your dog to "push!" When she does, toss a treat at the base of the ball.

4. Remove the training rails. Some dogs will get very excited and bite and pop the ball while learning. Always deliver your treat near the base of the ball to encourage your dog to poke under the ball instead of biting it.

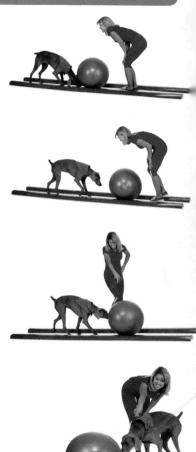

Paintbrush Painting

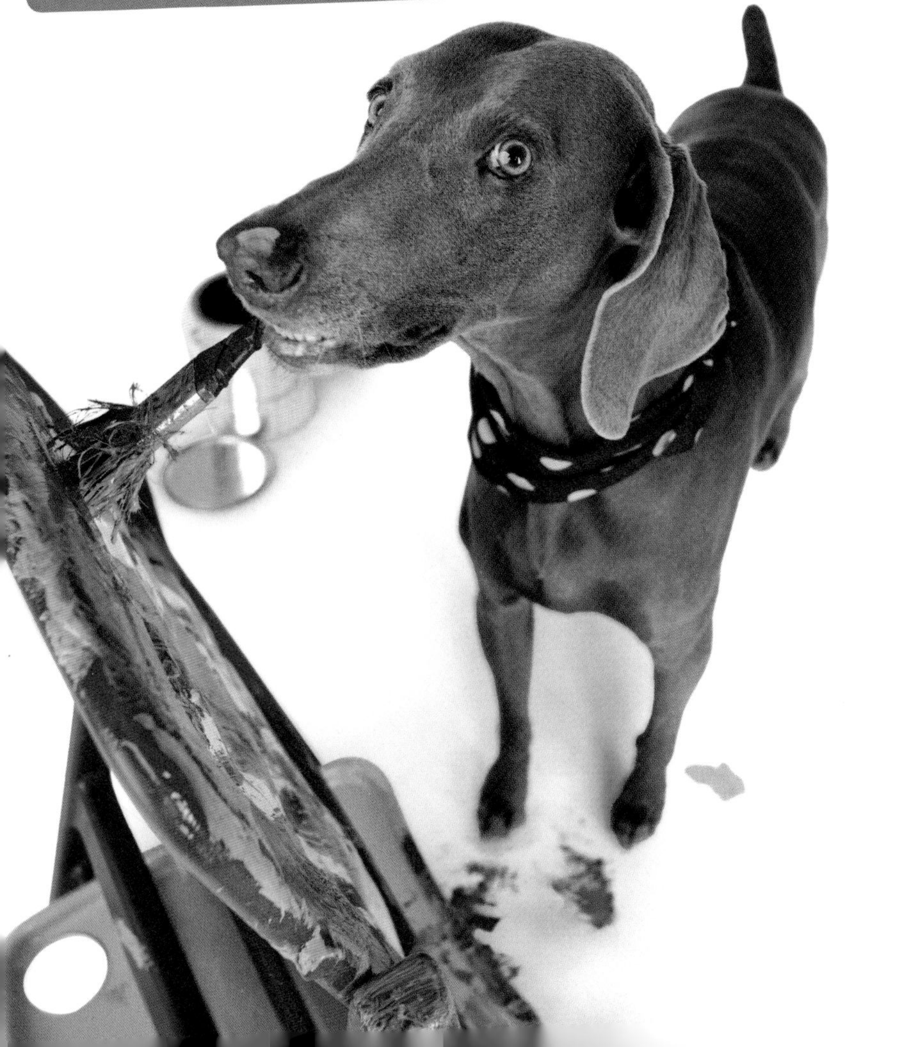

1. After teaching **touch my hand** (page 36), hold a paint can lid in your hand for your dog to nose-touch. You can put a dab of peanut butter on it.

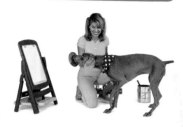

2. Tape or hold the lid against your easel. Say, "Touch!" and give your dog a treat for nose-touching it.

3. Remove the lid and instead make an **X** on the canvas with colored tape for your dog to touch.

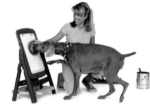

4. Hopefully your dog enjoys holding things in her mouth or has learned to **fetch** (page 188). Have her take the paintbrush in her mouth and cue her to nose-touch the canvas. Because the paintbrush extends in front of her, she will end up stabbing the brush into the canvas.

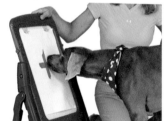

EQUIPMENT: Use nontoxic, washable kids' paint.

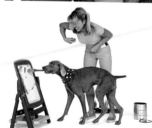

Come

Call your dog to "come" only for good things and never for bad things (such as a bath or nail trimming). This will keep him eager to come to you!

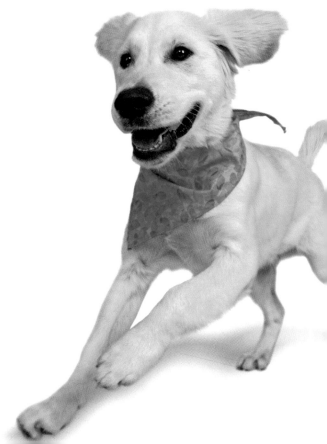

1. Pat your legs, open your arms, and call "come."

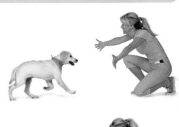

2. Reward your dog profusely when he reaches you.

3. Engage your dog's chase drive by calling "come" and running away from him. Remember, catching you is his reward, so make it fun!

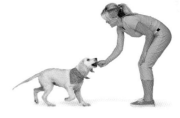

4. Put your dog on a lead and tell him to "come." If he does not come to you on his own, reel him in. In both cases, reward him when he gets to you.

TROUBLESHOOTING: Keep this command happy, and reward your dog every time he comes (with a treat, praise, or a petting). If your dog runs off, do not chase him as that would encourage him to play keep-away. Act interested in something on the ground, or toss a toy around to get him to return to you.

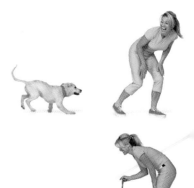

53

Dog Bowling

Call your dog through a narrow lane of bowling pins, and see who can get him to knock over the most pins. Strike!

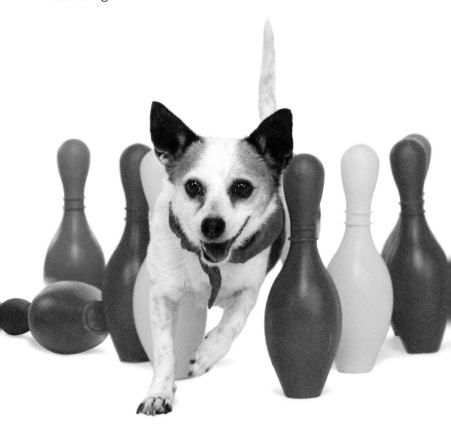

1. Set bowling pins (or plastic bottles) in a narrow hallway. Erect barriers, such as big boxes, on either side of the pins. Station one person at each end of the hall.

2. Call your dog to you so that he crashes through the bowling pins.

3. Give your dog a treat and count how many pins he knocked over. Reset the pins and have the other person call him. How many pins did he knock over this time?

TROUBLESHOOTING: Big, goofy dogs often crash right through the pins while smaller dogs may try to run between them. If your dog jumps over the pins, hold the treat close to the ground and not up high.

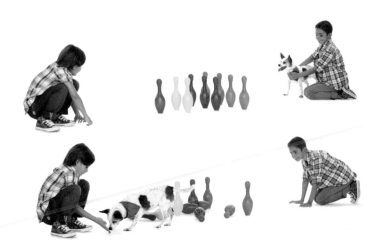

Messenger Dog

In this trick, your dog carries a top-secret message back and forth between two people, just like historic war dogs did.

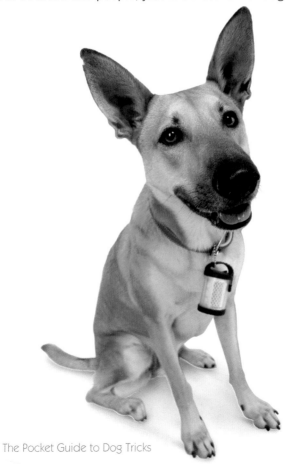

1. Have two people that your dog knows separate. Send the dog to the other person, saying, "Find [person's name]!"

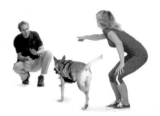

2. As the dog approaches him, the recipient should clap and encourage the dog. When the dog arrives, the recipient gives the dog enthusiastic praise or a treat.

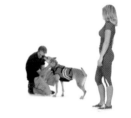

3. Now make it more difficult; have the person hold your dog while you run away and disappear around a corner. Can your dog still find you?

4. After you've sent your dog, take that opportunity to hide yourself in a new spot. Keep the game going, sending your dog back and forth between people.

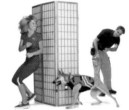

TIP! This is a great way to teach your dog each of your family member's names.

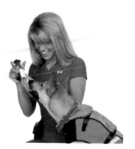

Back-Track to Your Toy

How good is your dog's memory? Challenge him to remember the location of his toy, and then go back to find it.

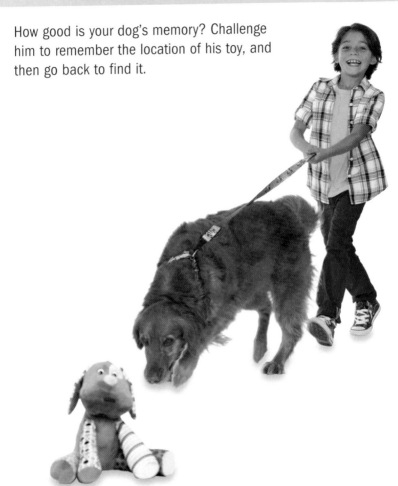

1. Show your dog his favorite toy (or food toy, or bowl with food in it) and set it on the ground. Point it out to him a few times and tell him to remember where it is.

2. Use a leash to walk him a short distance (about 30 feet, 10 meters) away from the toy.

3. Excitedly say, "Find it!" and maybe even point toward the toy. Let your dog run back to the toy or food bowl and get his reward. Next, place the toy in a new location and walk your dog farther away from the toy and try again.

WHAT TO EXPECT: Build distance gradually so your dog can be successful and won't get discouraged. Eventually, you may be able to backtrack a few hundred feet (meters).

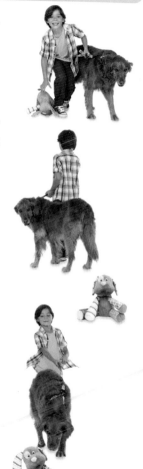

Scootering

This accessible sport is easy to learn and provides exercise for you and your dogs.

EQUIPMENT

Dog scooters are solidly constructed with off-road tires. The dog wears a mushing harness that is attached to the scooter by a tugline.

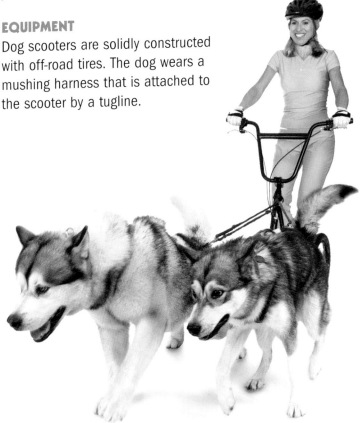

1. Attach a tugline to the back ring of your dog's harness. Set out your dog's food dish and tell him enthusiastically to "Hike!"

2. Attach the tugline to a box and try it again. The sound of the box moving may startle your dog at first. Stay behind your dog, as this will be your scootering position.

3. Finally, try it with your scooter. Keep your eye on the tugline so that it does not go slack and under your wheel.

TIP! Dogs run best in cool temperatures and in wilderness environments that are new and exciting to them. A dog will be more enthusiastic to run when competing against other dogs. Get some friends together and go scootering as a group.

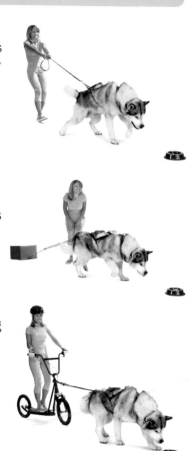

Leash Training (No Pulling)

Teach your dog to walk without pulling. Your dog wants to move forward. We will allow her to move forward only when she has a slack leash. When the leash is taut ... we stop.

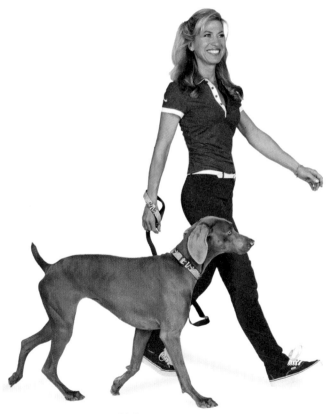

1. Start your walk with a slack leash.
2. As soon as your dog pulls ...
3. Stop in your tracks, and wait.
4. Eventually, the leash will go slack. As soon as the leash goes slack for one second, say "good" and continue your walk. There are no treats in this skill, as the walk *is* the reward.

WHAT TO EXPECT: The first time you attempt this method, you can expect to be stopped every few seconds. This is normal. It *will* get better. Few people have the patience to stick with this plan, but it is an extremely effective method once taught.

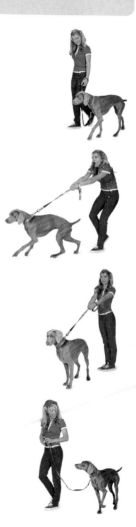

Bark the Answer

"Buddy, how old are you?" Ruff! Ruff! Ruff! "That's right, you're three!" Teach your dog to bark on cue.

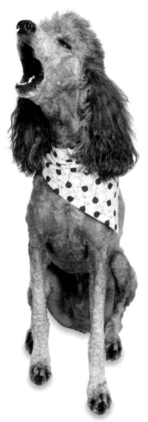

1. Most dogs bark at the sound of the doorbell. Stand at your front door with the door open (so your dog can hear the doorbell). Say "bark!" in a voice that kind of sounds like a bark, and press the doorbell.

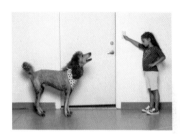

2. If your dog barks, say "good bark!" and give him a treat. Repeat this about six times.

3. On the seventh time, say "bark!" and pretend to ring the doorbell, but don't actually ring it. You may have to say "bark!" a few more times. If your dog barks, give him a treat! If he doesn't bark, go back to ringing the doorbell.

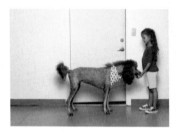

TROUBLESHOOTING: If your dog doesn't respond to the sound of the doorbell, try something else to get him to bark, such as a friend knocking on your door or tapping a window with a metal key.

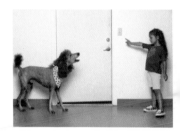

Paws Up

Teach your dog to put his front paws up onto a stool.

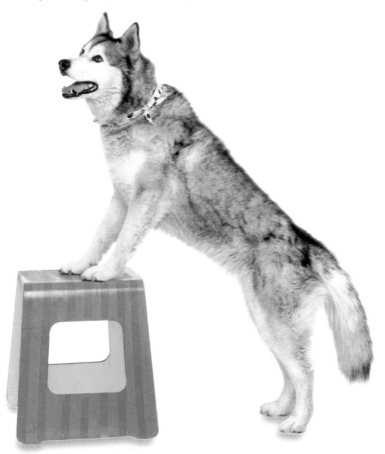

1. Slowly move a treat from your dog's nose up over the stool. Say, "Paws up!" and pat the stool to encourage him.

2. As he starts to reach for the treat, move it higher, just out of his reach. He'll step onto the stool to reach for the treat. Hold the treat still and don't move it away from him anymore.

3. When he reaches the treat, tell him "good!" and let him take the treat from your hand.

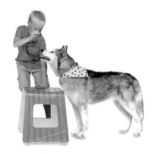

TROUBLESHOOTING: If your dog walks around the stool but won't step on it, or steps on it with only one paw, switch to a lower stool. If your dog is jumping over the stool entirely, move your hand slower when you lure him.

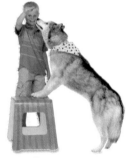

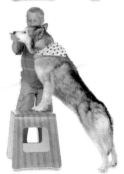

Paws on My Arm

If your pet peeve is a pet that jumps on guests, teach him to welcome visitors with **paws on their arm** to give him a safe and manageable way to show his enthusiasm.

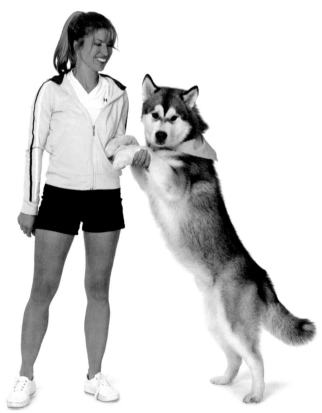

The Pocket Guide to Dog Tricks

1. Sit on the floor with your dog on your left. Raise your left arm and lure his head upward with a treat in your right hand. Your dog will probably place one or both paws on your forearm, in an effort to reach the treat, but if he doesn't, you can coax his paws onto your arm with your hands. Once your dog is in the correct position, with his paws resting on your arm, let him nibble treats from your hand.

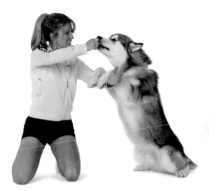

2. Try this trick while standing up. Position your arm perpendicular to your body and have your dog approach from the outside so as to prevent him from knocking you over or overextending your shoulder.

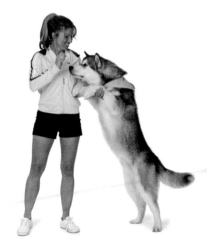

Push a Shopping Cart

Standing on his hind legs, your dog puts his paws up and pushes a shopping cart.

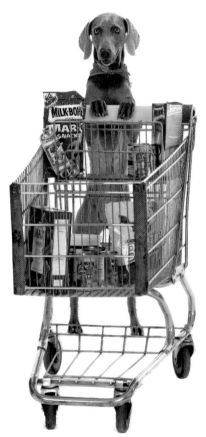

1. First teach **paws up** (page 66). Have your dog put her paws up on a bar. Slowly walk backward to get her used to moving.

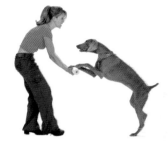

2. Lay a towel over the cart's grating to prevent your dog's paws from getting stuck. Tap the handle and tell her "paws up." Stand to the side of the cart and hold it to prevent it from rolling. Hold a treat in front of her and coax her forward. Reward your dog for her first steps.

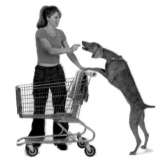

3. Stand at the opposite end of the cart and use a treat near your dog's nose to lure her forward.

TIP! A grassy surface works well for this trick, as it will slow the cart down. Keep control of the cart during the learning process, as a slip could cause significant setbacks.

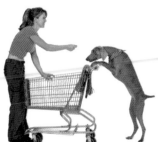

Say Your Prayers

In this trick, your dog bows her head between her paws like she is saying her prayers.

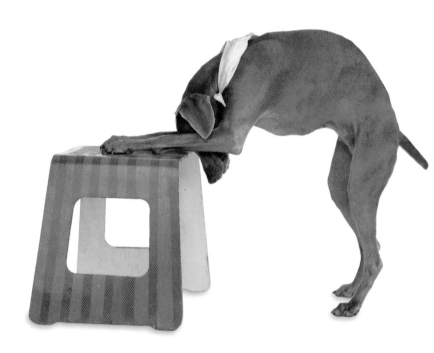

1. Hold several small treats in both hands. Stand to the side of your dog and hold one treat to her nose.

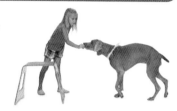

2. Say "paws up" and move the treat forward and up over the stool.

3. Let your dog nibble the treat from that hand.

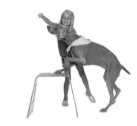

4. Say "prayers." Reach your other hand up from below your dog's chest, and slowly bring both of your hands together until they touch near your dog's front paws. Take away your first hand and try to get her to nibble treats from your lower hand.

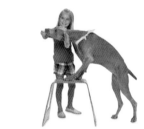

TROUBLESHOOTING: If your dog drops one paw off the stool, it may be that she is having a hard time reaching the treat. Hold the treat closer to her paws instead of her chest. Hold the treat in the center and not more toward one leg.

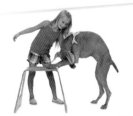

Turn on a Tap Light

It's getting dark ... send your helpful dog to step on a tap light.

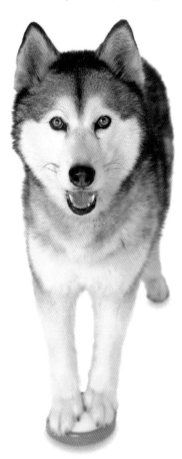

1. First, teach your dog to put his **paws up** on a stool (page 66). Now try a shorter stool.

2. Do paws up on a cement brick. Next, tape a tap light to the brick. Give your dog a treat for stepping on the brick. Give extra-excited praise if he happens to step on the tap light itself!

3. Tape the light to a smaller object, such as an upside-down dog bowl. Say "lights!" Give him a treat if he touches the tap light at all (even if it doesn't actually turn on).

4. Lay the tap light directly on the floor (tape it down if your dog scratches at it). If he has trouble, go back to the previous step.

WHAT TO EXPECT: You're going to be tempted to skip a few steps in this trick but it's best not to. Increase difficulty slowly by doing a paws up on just a slightly smaller object each time.

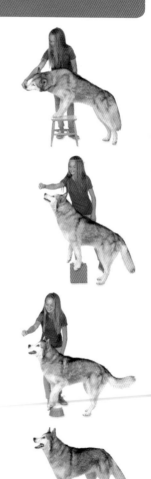

Teach your dog to fit all four paws on a small brick. Careful ... don't lose your balance!

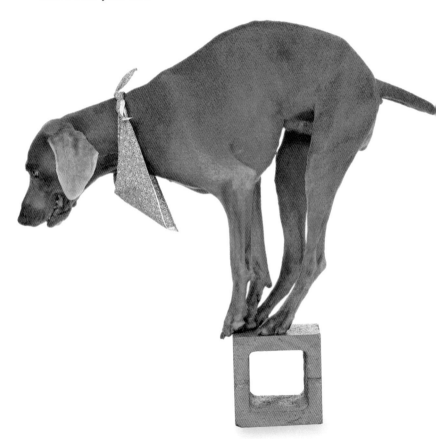

1. Arrange four bricks into a platform. Say "step up" and use your treat to lure her forward. When all four paws are on the platform, give her the treat.

2. Remove one brick. If you have trouble getting your dog's back feet on the bricks, keep moving the treat forward until your dog's front feet come off the bricks at the same time that her back feet come on. Give her a treat for that. This teaches her that the trick has something to do with her back feet.

3. Arrange two and a half bricks in a line, like a balance beam. This platform is narrower (which is harder than the last step), but also longer (which is easier). Stand to the side and move your treat in a straight line.

4. Once she is doing it well, take away a brick—and then another.

5. Finally, use just the small half brick.

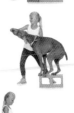

77

Ride in a Wagon

Pull your dog around the neighborhood in a wagon. What a buddy!

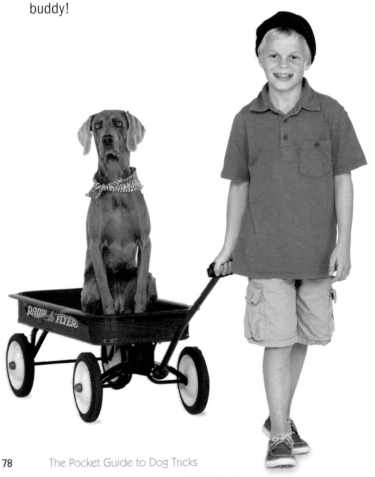

1. Wrap a towel around the wagon wheel to keep it from moving. Use several small treats to lure your dog to put her paws up into the wagon.

2. Continue moving your hand forward to encourage her to put her back feet up. When she is all the way in the wagon, give her another treat.

3. Keep giving her treats every few seconds to encourage her to stay in the wagon, as she will probably want to jump out.

4. Tell her to "stay," hold your hand up, and back up one step. Go back and give her a treat.

TROUBLESHOOTING: Put a doormat in the wagon to give your dog traction. For small dogs, put a cement brick next to the wagon as a step to help her get in. If your dog is scared, let her jump out if she needs to, but try to keep her in by feeding her treats.

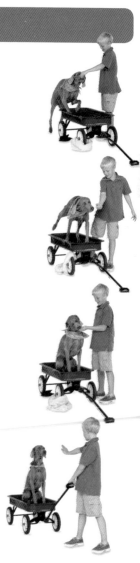

Spot Training

Teach your dog to go to her "spot" (her dog bed) and stay there. Take your "spot" with you on the road, to give your dog security in an unfamiliar place.

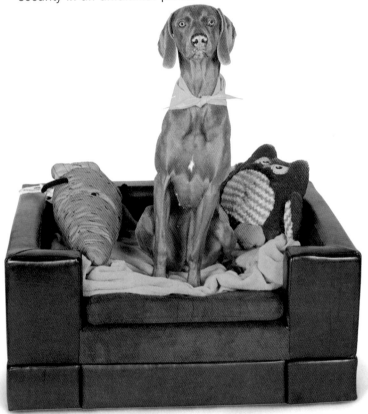

1. Say "go to your spot!" and toss a treat onto your dog's bed. Let her run to her bed and eat the treat.

2. Have her lie down in her bed (as she is more likely to stay there in a down position). Tell her "stay," and back up a few steps.

3. Go forward and reward her with a treat or praise. Build up farther distances and longer stays.

4. If your dog breaks her stay and leaves her spot, immediately send her back. Ideally you can direct her back without a treat, but if there is no other way, use a treat to lure her back onto her spot.

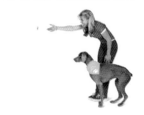

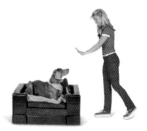

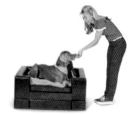

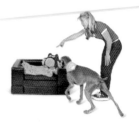

Kennel Up

Your dog needs a special crate or dog bed of his very own.
Teach him a name for his kennel so you can send him there for
bedtime.

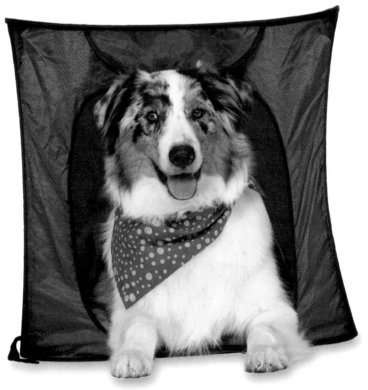

1. Toss a treat in your dog's crate as you tell him to "kennel up." Do this a couple of times a day for several days.

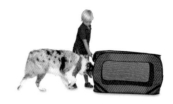

2. By now, he will be pretty excited to kennel up. This time, say "kennel up" and pretend to toss a treat into his kennel.

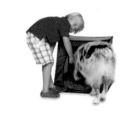

3. Once he goes in the crate, hand him a treat. Be sure to give the treat while he is still inside the crate.

4. As he gets better, you can stand farther away when you send him to his kennel. Then walk over and give him a treat in his crate.

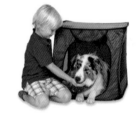

WHAT TO EXPECT: As part of his bedtime routine your dog will look forward to kenneling up and receiving his good night treat. Your dog's kennel is his personal place that he goes to when he wants to be left alone. Don't crawl into his kennel or reach inside.

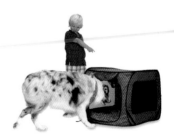

Surfing

Standing on a body board is not easy. Teach your dog slowly until he gains confidence and masters this wobbly toy. Never force or lift your dog into the water, as that will make him more fearful. It's better to take it slowly, even if it takes several sessions before your dog places his first paw in the water.

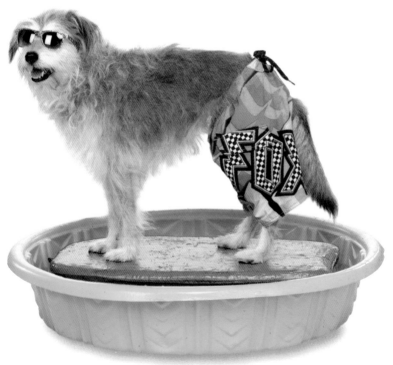

1. Introduce your dog to the body board on dry land. Use a treat to lure him onto it and let him nibble the treat while he has a paw on the board.

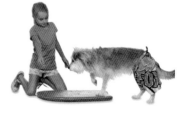

2. Put the body board in an empty wading pool. Again, use a treat to lure your dog to step on it and let him nibble the treat there.

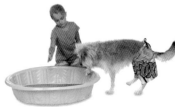

3. Fill the wading pool with just a few inches (5 cm) of water and lure your dog with a treat just as you did before. Use your foot to stabilize the board.

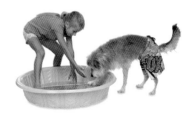

4. Fill the pool with more water. Encourage your dog to jump onto the board and make a splash! If he's having fun, he'll be more confident.

TROUBLESHOOTING: If your dog is skittish of the plastic surface, put an inch (2 cm) of sand in the bottom of the pool.

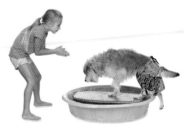

Skateboard

Your dog can learn to push a skateboard by placing three paws on top and pushing with her remaining back paw.

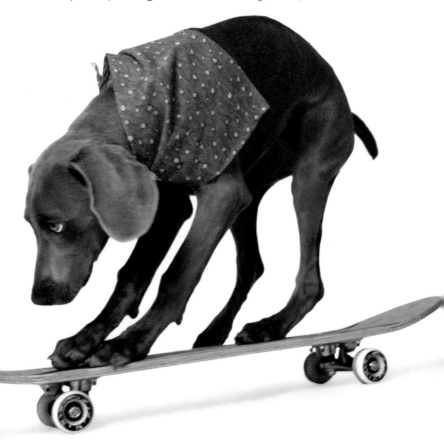

1. Hold the skateboard still with your foot, and lure your dog to put her **paws up** (page 66). The moment her paws come up on the skateboard, give her the treat.

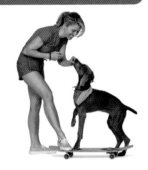

2. Now teach her to put a third paw on the skateboard. Hold a treat near your dog's nose to keep her head and front paws in place. Tap her rear leg which is closest to the skateboard to give her the idea to move it onto the skateboard. When she does, give her the treat.

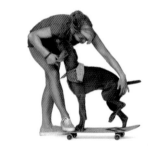

3. It's time to get rolling. Attach a leash around the front wheels. Have your dog put three paws on the skateboard, and keep her attention by holding a treat slightly ahead of her. Pull very slowly on the leash. The instant her fourth paw leaves the ground, say "good!" and give her a treat. Continue pulling and treating.

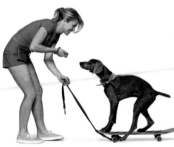

Fit Ball

Improve your dog's balance, strength, and coordination by having her balance on top of a wobbly fit ball.

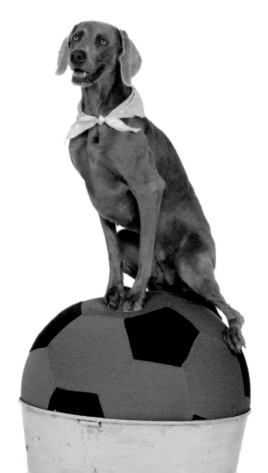

1. Use a box or bucket to stabilize your fit ball. Move a treat from your dog's nose over the ball to get her to put her paws up. Let her nibble treats in your hand to keep her there. Gently rock the ball back and forth so she uses her rear legs to balance.

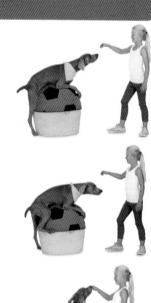

2. Move the treat just out of your dog's reach to coax her to climb on top of the ball. She will try to move around the ball. Keep moving your body so the ball is between you and your dog.

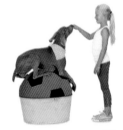

3. Give your dog treats as long as she is trying, even if she can't quite get on top of the ball. If she does get on the ball, let her nibble treats from your hand and lean against your hand for balance.

4. Once your dog is feeling comfortable, walk slowly around the ball so she has to stand up to follow your treats.

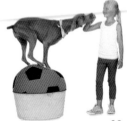

Barrel

Rolling a barrel will be challenging for your dog as she learns to control her balance and place her feet deliberately.

EQUIPMENT
Construct a barrel from a 55-gallon (208 L) plastic drum (sold at horse feed stores.) Cover the barrel with rubber mat or carpet.

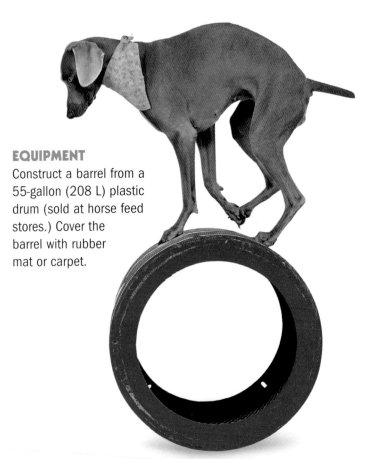

1. Place the barrel against a wall or use your hand to hold it still. Hold a treat above the barrel to lure your dog to put his paws up. Encourage him to stay there by giving him small treats every few seconds.

2. Hold a treat in front of your dog to keep his attention and use your other hand to roll the barrel away from your dog a few inches. Every time he repositions a paw, say, "Good!" and give him a treat.

3. Stand on the opposite side of the barrel and hold it with your knee or foot. Use a handful of treats to lure your dog on top of the barrel. As he tries to steady himself he may press against your hand, which is fine.

4. Very slowly, roll the barrel a few inches backward, so that your dog has to take a step forward. Keep your hand with the treats by his nose and give him a treat every few seconds.

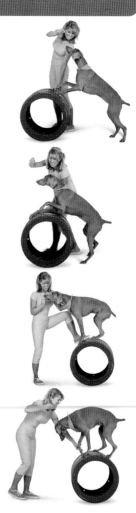

Climb a Ladder

Climbing a ladder requires not only coordination and strength but also confidence.

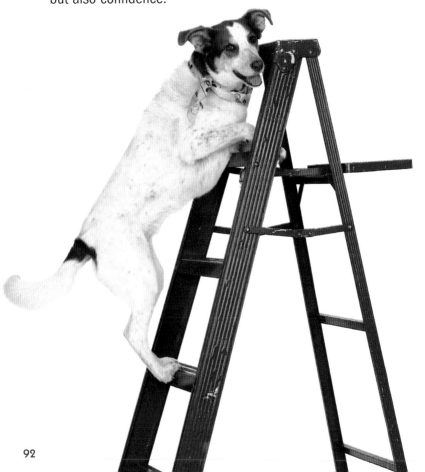

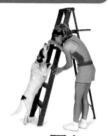

1. Cover the steps of a sturdy ladder with a nonslip surface. Using a treat, lure your dog to place his paws up on a rung. Do not touch or confine your dog, as he will want to feel he has an escape route. Raise the treat higher.

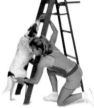

2. Still luring your dog's head upward, use your other hand to coax his back paw onto the first step.

3. Your dog is now in a precarious position, so guard his body to stabilize him. Continue to raise the treat and allow him to position his front paws himself.

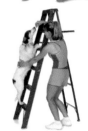

4. Once your dog is comfortable climbing the steps, place your treat at the top of the ladder to motivate a speedy ascent!

WHAT TO EXPECT: Regardless of your dog's athletic ability, you should lift him to the floor rather than letting him jump down, as there is potential for injury due to his twisting motion or entanglement in the ladder rungs.

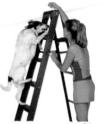

Muffin Tin

Hide tiny treats in a muffin tin and cover the cups with tennis balls. Can your dog figure out how to get the treats?

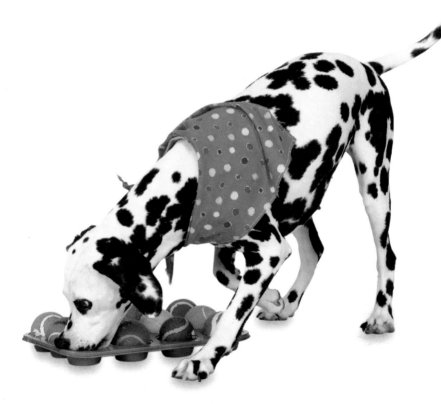

1. Let your dog watch as you place one treat in each muffin tin cup.

2. Tell your dog excitedly to "find it!" and let him come eat the treats.

3. Try the same thing again, only this time place a tennis ball in one of the cups (on top of a treat). Encourage your dog to get all of the treats, including the one under the ball.

4. The next time, put treats in all the cups and cover half of them with tennis balls. Can your dog find all of the treats?

TROUBLESHOOTING: If your dog gives up, lift one of the tennis balls to show him the treat underneath.

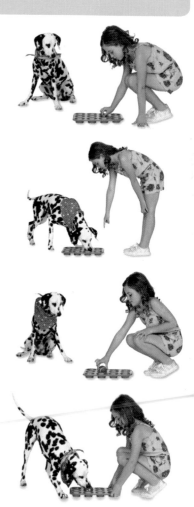

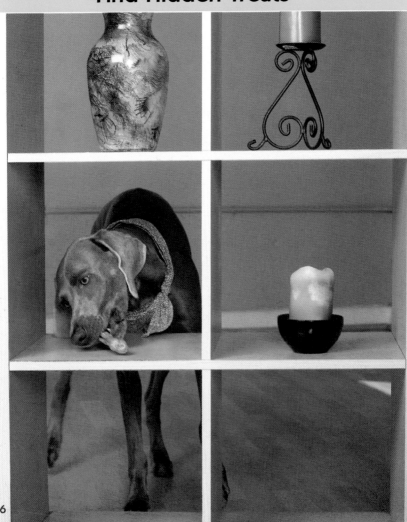

Hide treats around the house and watch your dog sleuth them out. Bet she can find them all!

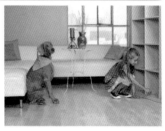

1. Tell your dog to "stay"or have someone hold her collar. Hide a treat in a really easy spot, just a few feet from her, on or near the floor.

2. Say "find it!" and point to the treat.

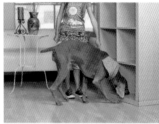

3. Try it again, but this time hide the treat in a harder spot, like up off the floor. Don't make it too hard yet though.

4. As your dog improves, hide the treats under cushions, behind doors, or even in other rooms. Have your dog wait while you run around the house and hide a whole bunch of treats.

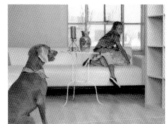

TROUBLESHOOTING: Use small treats like dog kibble, goldfish crackers, popcorn, cheese puffs, or "Cheerios" cereal.

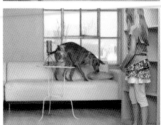

Search in Ball Pit

Even dogs think it's fun to jump in a ball pit! Hide a treat or toy in a bucket full of balls and watch your dog dive in after it. Instead of balls, you can also use crumpled newspaper balls.

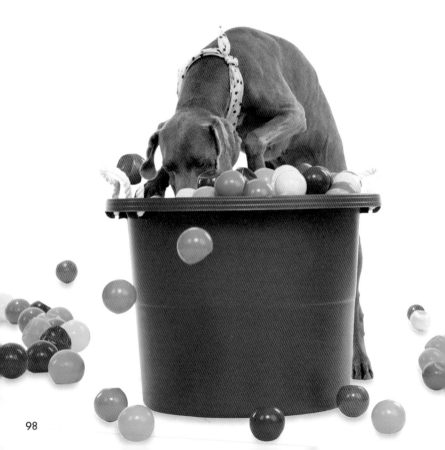

1. You'll need a smelly food toy like a chewable bone, a peanut butter–filled toy, or even a baggie filled with treats. Show your dog the bone to get her interest, and lay it right on top of the balls. Tell her to "get it!"

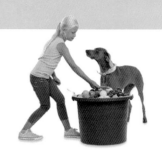

2. When she finds the bone, let her play with it for a while as a reward.

3. Bury the bone a little deeper (but not too deep).

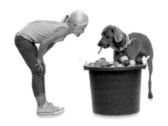

4. Your dog will have to hunt for it this time. Where did it go? Can she find it?

WHAT TO EXPECT: Some dogs are cautious about putting their head under all of those balls, but they usually gain confidence over time. Don't make it too hard for your dog too fast. Bury the bone just a little deeper each time.

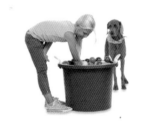

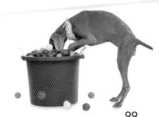

Laundry Basket

Does your dog have a favorite toy or food treat? Hide it under a laundry basket. He can see the toy, and smell the toy, but can't get the toy. Challenge him to solve this puzzle.

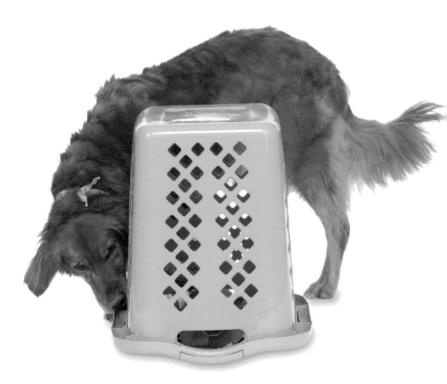

1. Show your dog as you put his favorite bone or toy under a laundry basket. Let him poke around at it for ten seconds, and then tilt it up so he can squeeze under and get his toy. Now we've got him interested in this game!

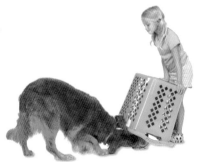

2. Try the game again, only this time let your dog struggle with it a little longer before you help him. We want him to eventually figure it out on his own.

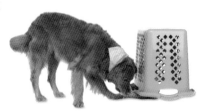

TROUBLESHOOTING: If your dog gives up, make sure you've got something he really wants under the laundry basket (usually food!) Try a peanut butter–filled toy or a chewable dog bone.

Bread Crumb Trail

Drop a trail of treats through your yard. Can your dog follow the path and find the treasure at the end?

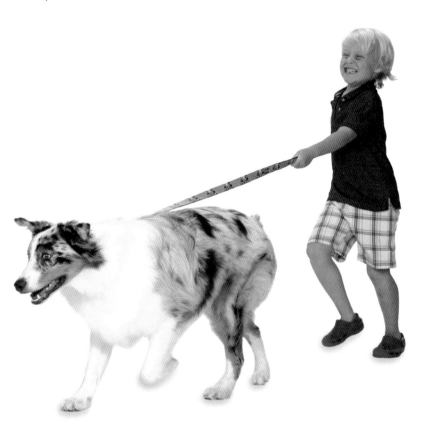

1. Lay a line of treats through your yard, or down a path. Use rather large treats that your dog can see, such as popcorn. Put them a few feet apart. Put a treasure at the end, like a special dog bone or toy.

2. Leash your dog and show him the first treat. Let him sniff out the path. As he starts to find more treats, he'll get more excited and pull you along. Did he find the treasure at the end?

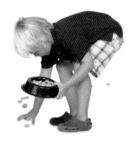

TROUBLESHOOTING: This is a fun and simple game for any dog. Some dogs can get quite excited to find the treats and will pull on their leash. If your dog is having trouble staying on the path, put the treats closer together or try using smellier treats (liver and salmon treats are pretty smelly).

Guess Which Hand

Hide a treat in one hand and ask your dog to "Guess which hand?" If she gets it right, she gets the treat!

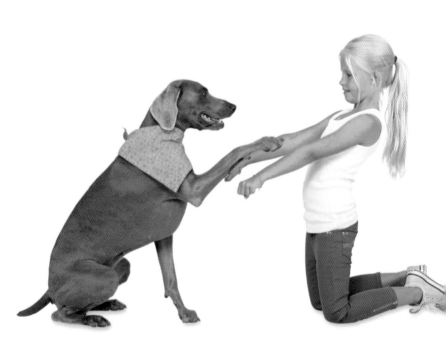

1. Hold a treat in one fist (but not too tightly, so your dog can still smell it). Hold out both fists to your dog and ask "Which hand?"

2. Your dog will probably sniff both of your hands, and then decide which one she thinks has the treat. She'll then sniff that hand more, and may even paw at it.

3. If she chose correctly, say, "Good!" and open your hand to let her have the treat.

4. If your dog chose incorrectly, open the hand she chose to show her that it is empty. Then try the game again.

WHAT TO EXPECT: Dogs usually enjoy this game and catch on quickly.

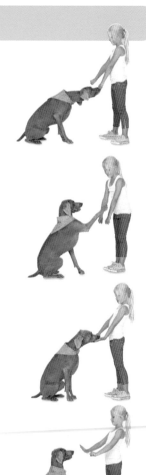

Nose Work Box Search

In this nose-work game, the dog sniffs boxes to find the one containing a target scent.

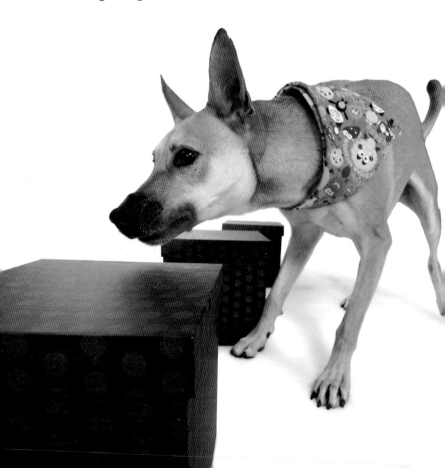

1. Set out three to six open boxes. Put some strong-smelling treats in a ventilated container (so your dog can't eat them). Hide the treat container in one of the boxes.

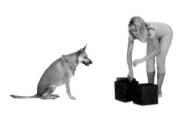

2. Release your dog to search for the "hide." Don't say anything while your dog searches, as it will distract him. If your dog needs encouragement, nonchalantly investigate the boxes yourself.

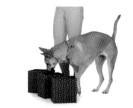

3. When your dog shows interest in the correct box, enthusiastically praise him and give him a treat. (Give the treat next to the correct box.)

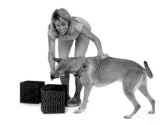

4. Increase the difficulty by partially closing the boxes. Punch holes in the boxes for ventilation, so your dog can smell the treats inside.

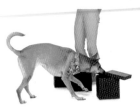

Shell Game

In this classic game, a ball is placed beneath one of three cups. The cups are shuffled and your dog shows you which one is hiding the ball. (The secret to this game is in the scent!)

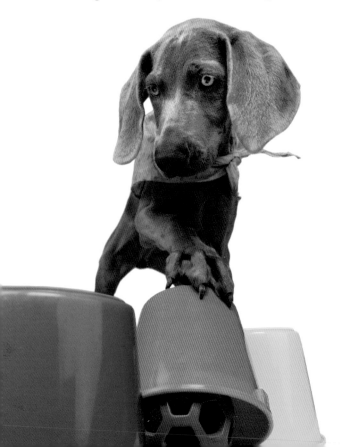

EQUIPMENT

Use plastic or clay flower pots which have a hole in the bottom. Your dog will use this hole to smell the treat.

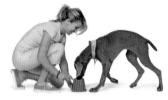

1. Use a strong smelling treat, such as beef jerky. Let your dog sniff it, and then put it under a game cup.

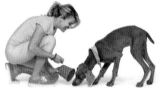

2. When she shows interest, say "good!," lift the cup and let her get the treat. If she loses interest, lift the cup to reveal the treat and put it down again.

3. Add more cups. If she sniffs or paws an incorrect cup, hold the cup in place and encourage her to keep looking.

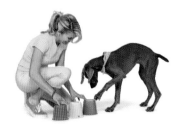

4. When she shows interest in the correct cup, lift it up.

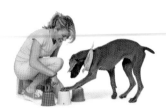

Bobbing for Popcorn

This is a great game to play with your dog on a hot summer day. Teach him to become comfortable in water by having him pick out popcorn from a shallow pool. Go ahead, dive right in!

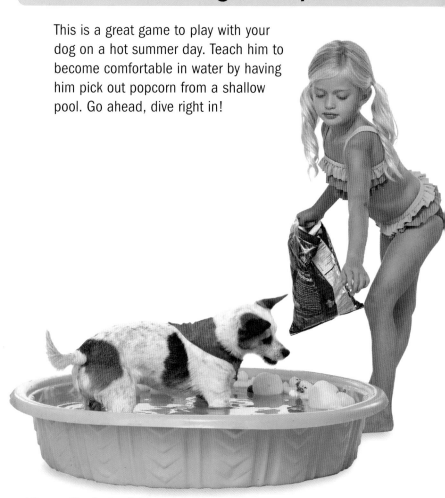

1. Sit in an empty wading pool and hold out some popcorn to your dog. He may be unsure about the wading pool and need a little time to get used to it before he is confident enough to step inside.

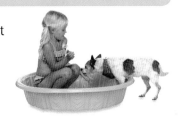

2. Put just an inch (2 cm) of water in the pool. Move your treat to the middle of the pool to try to get your dog to step inside. Put a little more water in the pool. Toss some popcorn in the water. Your dog will try to get the popcorn, but may be hesitant to step all the way inside. That's okay, give him time to get used to it.

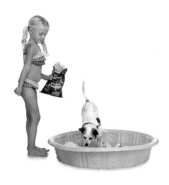

3. Fill the pool to the top. Sprinkle popcorn in the pool and let your dog have fun finding them and fishing them out.

TROUBLESHOOTING: Some dogs love water and some do not. Never lift your dog into the pool; let him decide on his own when he is ready to enter.

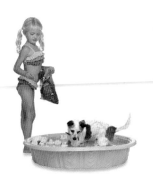

Wipe Your Paws

When it's muddy outside, you'll be glad you taught your dog to wipe his paws on a doormat!

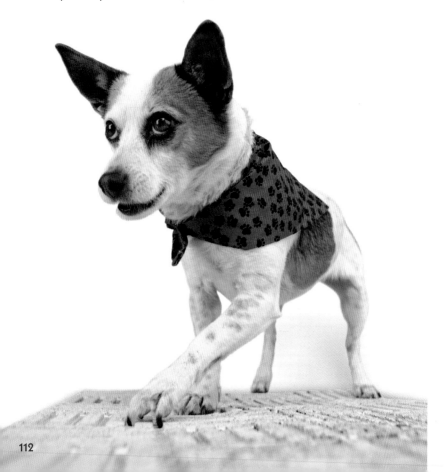

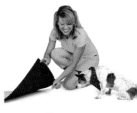

1. Show your dog as you put a treat on the ground (hard dog biscuits work best). Cover the treat with the doormat, so that the treat is near the corner of the mat.

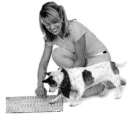

2. Hold the edge of the doormat down in case your dog tries to poke his nose under it. Encourage him to "Get it! Get it!" If he loses interest, lift the corner of the doormat quickly to show him the treat.

3. When he gets frustrated, your dog will scratch at the doormat—be ready for this! Say, "Good!" and lift the doormat for him to get the treat.

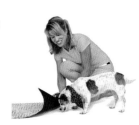

4. As he improves, you can then stop putting the treat under the doormat and toss it where he is digging instead (it will be more fun for him to "dig up" the treat rather than getting it from your hand).

WHAT TO EXPECT: Dogs usually nose the doormat a lot at first and might do just one tentative scratch—don't miss it! Reward your dog for just the slightest scratch.

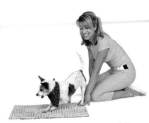

Down

Teach your dog to lie down.

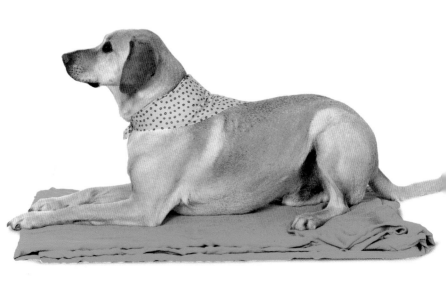

1. Hold a treat to his nose.

2. Lower the treat slowly to the floor. It can help to have your dog backed up to a wall. If your dog slouches instead of lying down, slide the treat slowly toward him on the floor between his front paws...

3. ... or slide the treat away from him. Release the treat once your dog lies down.

4. Once your dog is consistently lying down, gradually delay the release of the treat. With your dog lying down, say "wait, wait" and then "good" and release the treat. Varying the time before treating will keep your dog focused.

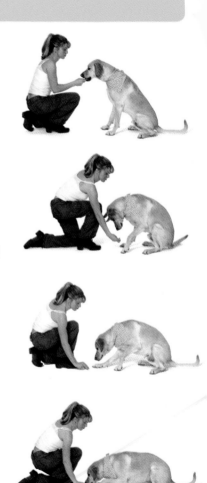

Play Dead

When playing dead, your dog rolls onto his back and lies still.

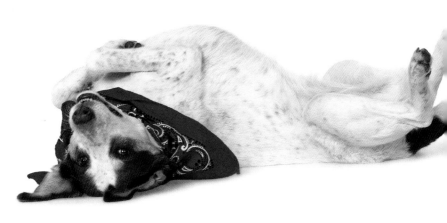

1. Put your dog in a **down** (page 114) and kneel in front of him.

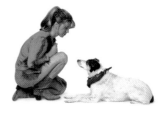

2. Hold a treat to the side of his head and move it toward his shoulder blade. Your dog should flop on to his side.

3. Continue to roll him to his back by moving the treat toward his backbone. Praise him and give him a belly scratch while he is on his back.

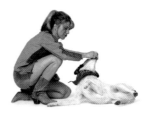

4. Give your dog the cue of "bang!" while he is upside down.

WHAT TO EXPECT: This position can be a little awkward for your dog, and will take some getting used to.

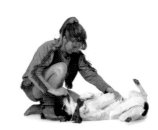

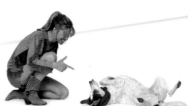

Roll Over

Small breed dogs sometimes have an easier time rolling over, but all dogs are capable of learning this trick. This trick will be harder for stocky dogs with short necks, such as bulldogs.

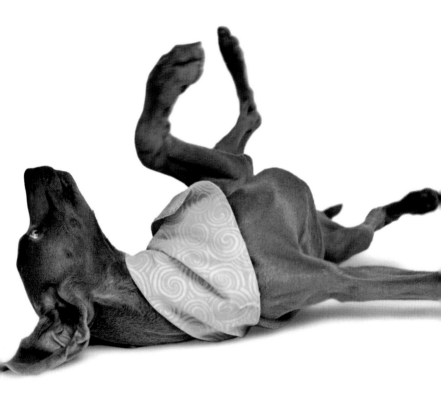

1. Hold several treats in your hand. Move your hand from your dog's nose to the side of her head.

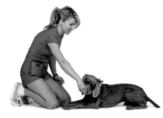

2. Continue to move the treats toward her shoulder blade. When your dog flops onto her side, release one treat.

3. Continue to move the treats from her shoulder blade toward her backbone. This should lure her to roll onto her back.

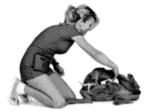

4. Keep going until she lands on her other side, and give her another treat.

TIP! It often helps to lean your body in the direction of the roll over, to influence your dog in that direction. Feel free to give multiple treats along the way, to keep your dog engaged in the rollover.

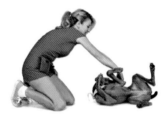

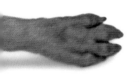

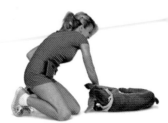

Take a Bow

Your dog **bows** by keeping his back legs upright, while bowing down his front until his elbows touch the floor.

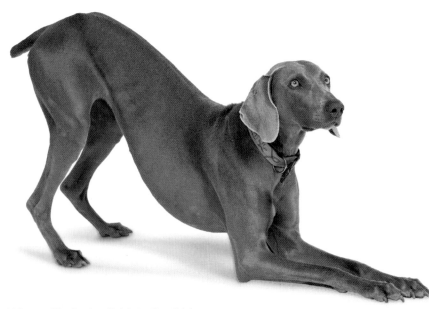

1. Hold a treat in your fist at nose height.

2. Press your hand into your dog's nose and downward, as if you are pressing toward his rear paws.

3. As soon as your dog's elbows touch the floor, release the treat and back your hand away.

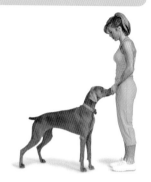

TROUBLESHOOTING: If your dog is sitting down instead of bowing, you are probably holding the treat to high.

If your dog is lying down, you need to release the treat sooner. You may have to release the treat before his elbows even touch the ground. If this does not solve the problem, position your foot on the floor under his belly.

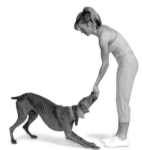

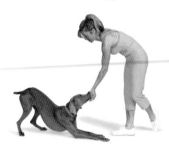

Spin Circles

Your dog **spins** either a left or a right full circle.

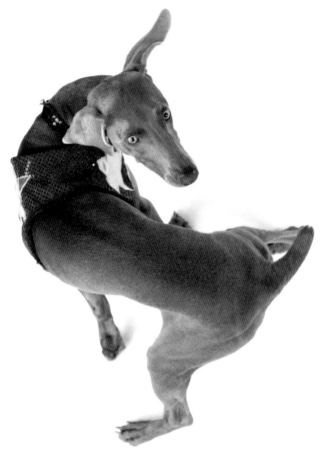

1. Begin with your dog facing you. Hold several treats in your right hand. Move your right hand to your right.

2. Continue to lure your dog in a large counter-clockwise circle. You may need to release a treat or two along the way, to keep your dog following your hand.

3. At the end of the circle, release the treat.

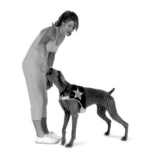

WHAT TO EXPECT: Dogs learn the spin trick easily. As she improves, diminish your hand signal until it is merely a flick of your wrist. Try it in the other direction; hold treats in your left hand and circle it in a clockwise direction.

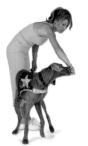

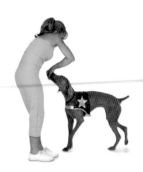

Balance Beam

Can your dog walk across a balance beam like a gymnast?
With a little help from you, I'll bet she can!

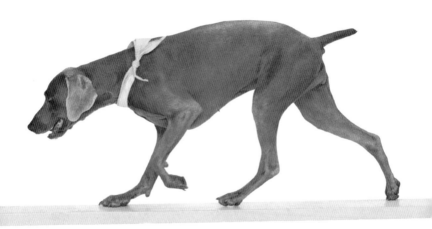

1. A picnic bench makes a wide, stable balance beam. (Little dogs may need a stepping stool to help them up.) Hold a treat to your dog's nose and move it slowly over the bench to get her to put her front paws up.

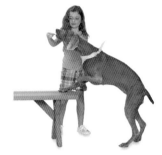

2. Continue to slowly move your treat forward, drawing your dog along.

3. Once she is up, slowly move your hand forward. Keep your hand low so your dog can still see the beam while watching your treat. Give her a treat every few steps. Give her a treat at the end, before she jumps off. Do not give treats after she has jumped off (or your dog will think she got a treat for being *off* the beam).

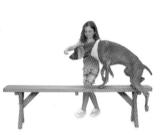

TIP! Put the bench alongside a wall to prevent her from jumping off. Use your body to block her.

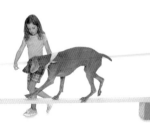

Double Balance Beam

The balance beam trick is doubly impressive when your dog walks on *two* skinny beams! Two paws walk on each rail.

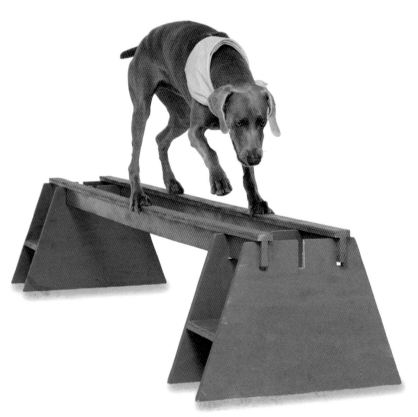

1. Teach your dog to walk a **balance beam** (page 124).

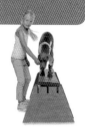

2. Replace the balance beam with two narrow beams pressed together. Use a treat to lure your dog all the way across. Keep the treat low, near the beams.

3. Arrange the beams in a V shape, with the "start" ends pressed together and the "finish" ends slightly separated. This V will force your dog to look down and think about her foot placement.

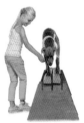

4. Finally, make both beams parallel and separated shoulder-width apart. Use a treat or your pointed finger to keep your dog going slow and straight.

TROUBLESHOOTING: We don't want your dog to get in the habit of jumping off in the middle. Give your dog a steady stream of treats going forward. Hold the treats low, near the beam.

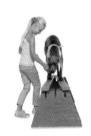

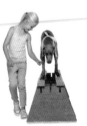

Build a Double Beam

SUPPLIES:

- 4 cement bond beam blocks: 8" × 8" × 16" (21.5 × 21.5 × 44 cm)
- 4 cement solid block caps: 2" × 8" × 16" (5 × 21.5 × 44 cm)
- 2 wood 2" × 4" studs (5 × 10 cm)
- Cement glue (optional)

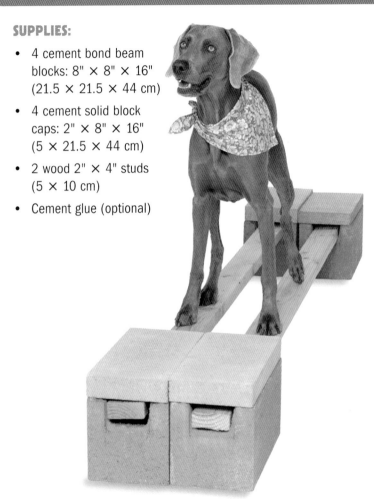

1. Set four cement bricks on a sturdy surface, with the grooves lining up. Push them snugly together. Place the wood beams in the grooves and adjust the placement of the bricks to the right distance apart.

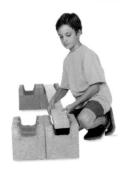

2. Squirt cement glue into the groove and squish the board down into it.

3. Place the caps on top of the bricks and secure with cement glue.

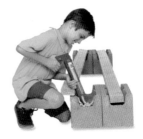

TIP! Enhance your double beam with paint and skid tape to improve traction.

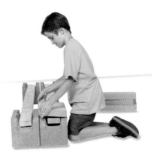

Teeter-Totter

Dogs who compete in the sport of agility learn to run across a teeter-totter. Your dog can learn it, too! The "bang" sound is scary for some dogs. With your dog off-leash, show him how the teeter-totter moves and let it bang quietly a few times.

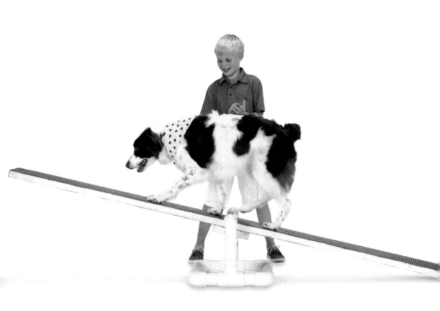

1. Set a box under each end of your teeter-totter. Hold a treat in front of your dog's nose, and guide him onto the board.

2. Slowly move your treat across the board. Hold the treat low so that your dog can still see the board while sniffing the treat.

3. Remove the box at the starting end of the teeter-totter.

4. Move slowly as you approach the middle of the board, when it is just about to fall.

5. Once your dog is crossing easily, remove the last box. If your dog is having problems, go back a step for a while.

TROUBLESHOOTING: If your dog is scared to go past the middle of the teeter-totter, place treats on the board just an inch (2 cm) out of his reach. If your dog is jumping off the middle of the teeter-totter, place it alongside a wall so he can't jump off that side.

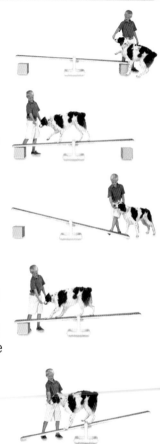

Build a Teeter-Totter

This simple teeter totter board rests on a base, making it easy to dismantle for travel or storage.

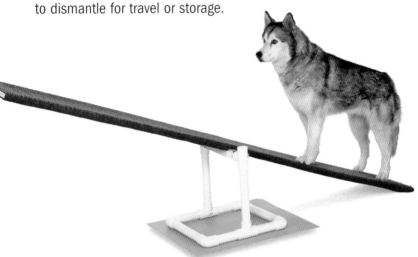

1. **Base:** Cut PVC pipe. Assemble the pieces together as shown.

2. **Stanchion:** Shorter uprights will make a shorter teeter.

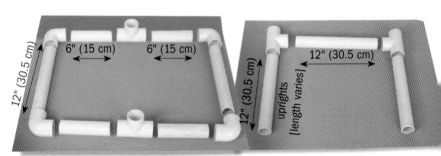

12" (30.5 cm)

6" (15 cm)   6" (15 cm)

12" (30.5 cm)

12" (30.5 cm)

uprights [length varies]

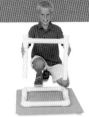

1. Fit the stanchion into the base.

2. **Build the board.** Glue two wood blocks parallel, in the center of your board. Leave enough space between them to fit a PVC T-joint.

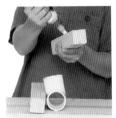

3. Put in several screws. Screw first into the board and down into the block.

4. Add traction by attaching outdoor turf or carpet to your board using a staple gun. Lay the board on top of the base, with the wood beams straddling the base crossbar.

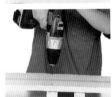

SUPPLIES

- PVC pipe (1¼")(3.2 cm)
- 4 PVC elbows (1¼")(3.2 cm)
- 4 PVC T-joints (1¼")(3.2 cm)
- Board (8'×1'×1")(2.4 m × 2.5 cm × 2.5 cm)
- Two wood blocks
  (2" × 2" × 12")(5 cm × 5 cm × 30.5 cm)
- Outdoor turf or carpet for traction
  (8' × 2')(2.4 m × 5 cm)
- Wood glue
- PVC cutting tool or saw
- Screws and screwdriver
- Staple gun

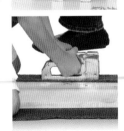

Handstand

Teach your dog to back up onto a ramp. Different dog breeds have different muscle structures, and some will be able to climb higher than others.

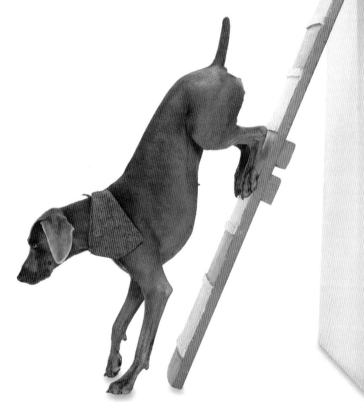

1. Push a treat slowly toward your dog's nose to get her to back up. When her back foot touches the board, say "good!" and release the treat. It's going to be tricky to keep moving your treat in such a way to get your dog to back up onto the board. Keep experimenting, and you'll get there.

2. Raise the board a little. Keep pushing the treat toward her to get her to take additional steps backward. Give her treats every few seconds as long as her feet remain on the board.

3. Raise the board higher. Put your hand low to the ground to keep her nose in the right position.

4. Lean the board against the wall to make it even higher. Your hand will now have to be almost at the floor.

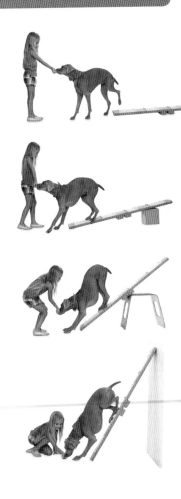

Sit

Sit is often the first trick a dog learns, and puppies as young as eight weeks old can learn this trick.

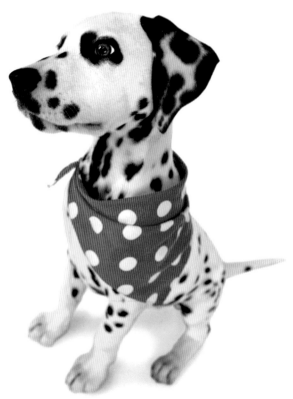

1. Hold a treat in front of your dog's nose. Say "sit" and slowly move the treat in an arc, up and back over her head. This should cause her nose to point up and her rear to drop.

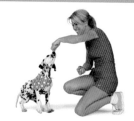

2. The instant her rear touches the floor, say "good!" and release the treat.

3. If your dog is jumping, it may be that you are holding your treat too high.

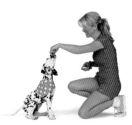

4. If your dog keeps moving backward instead of sitting, it may be that you are moving the the treat horizontally, instead of in an arc. Working with your dog in front of a wall will help, as your dog won't have room to move backward.

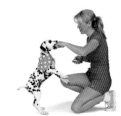

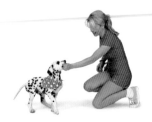

Sit Before Chowtime

It's never too early to start learning manners. Teach your polite pooch to sit before receiving his dinner. This will build a habit of your dog asking politely for his dinner.

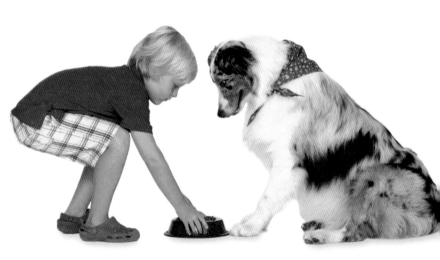

1. At mealtime, prepare your dog's bowl and tell him to "sit." He may be so excited that he temporarily forgets the meaning of the word, so give him several chances. Help him to sit by lifting the food bowl a little over his head and moving it toward him, which will cause his head to look up and his rear to drop.

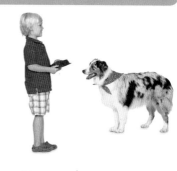

2. If he does not sit, turn away and put the bowl out of his reach. Come back in one minute and try again.

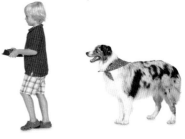

3. Try again a minute later. When your dog does finally sit, even for a second, say "good!" and put his bowl down as a reward for his politeness.

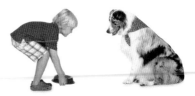

Stay

Sometimes, you need your dog to stay still.

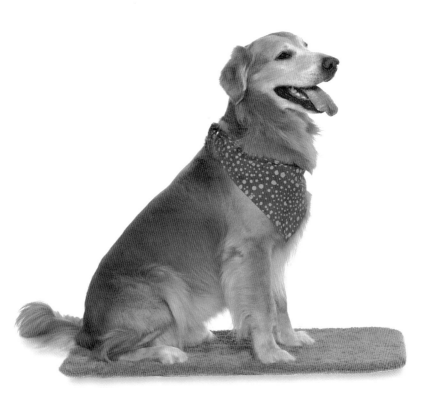

1. Stand in front of your dog. Raise your palm in front of his nose and say "stay" in a firm voice.

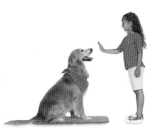

2. Keep your hand up as you take one step backward. Look into your dog's eyes to hold him in place. Act calm and use slow, deliberate movements.

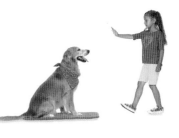

3. Wait one second, then step forward and give your dog a treat with your other hand (keep your first hand up until he has the treat). Give the treat only while your dog is sitting. Don't get the treat out of your pocket until you are standing in front of him, as the treat will pull him forward.

TROUBLESHOOTING: Gradually increase the time you ask your dog to stay, as well as the distance between you. You want your dog to be successful, so if he is standing up, go back to making it easier.

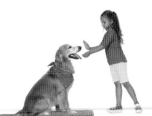

Watch Me

When you have your dog's eyes, you have his attention. Teach your dog to look directly into your eyes as a way to ask for his attention.

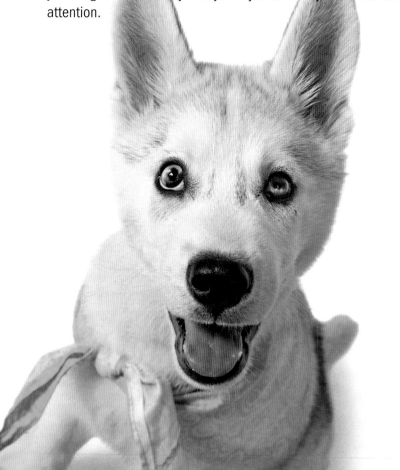

1. Get your dog's attention with a treat.

2. Bring the treat back toward your eyes, while saying "focus ... focus ... "

3. Once your dog holds eye contact for a second or two, say "good", and give him the treat. Build up time.

4. Phase out the handheld treat and instead use your pointed finger between your eyes and the word "focus" to cue his stare.

WHAT TO EXPECT: Shy dogs may be hesitant to look into your eyes, possibly because they feel it is confrontational. This exercise will be especially helpful for those timid dogs.

TIP! Make a habit of requiring a moment of calm attention before routine rewards, such as at the front door before a walk, or at the food dish before chowtime. This will teach your dog that calm, attentive behavior is rewarded.

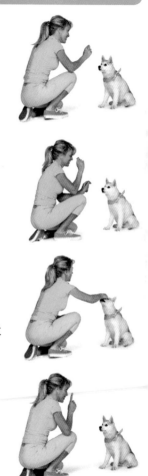

Balance and Catch

Your dog balances a treat or toy placed on his nose.

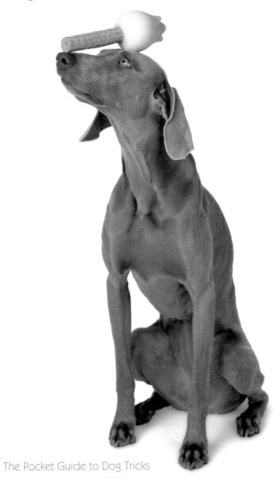

1. Gently hold your dog's muzzle parallel to the floor and place a treat upon the bridge of his nose. In a low voice, coach him to "waaaait."

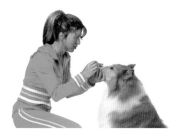

2. Hold this position for a few seconds before releasing his muzzle and telling him to "catch!" If your dog is allowing the treat to fall to the floor instead of attempting to catch it, pretend to race him to pick it up.

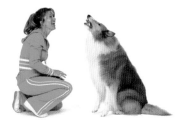

3. As your dog improves, require him to balance the treat on his nose without the help of your hand on his muzzle. Placing the treat near the end of your dog's nose is usually easiest to catch, but every dog is different.

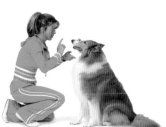

Memory Game

Hmmm ... now which one had the treat? This game is excellent training for a dog's focus and memory.

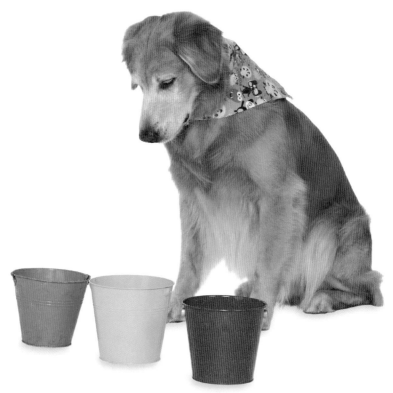

1. Set out two identical pails a few feet (60 cm) apart. Tell your dog to stay or have someone hold his collar.

2. Show your dog as you put a treat into one pail.

3. Tell him to "find it!" If he goes to the correct pail, he gets to eat the treat! If he goes first to the wrong pail, don't allow him to then check the other pail. Instead, put him back in a sit-stay and start all over.

4. Ready to make it harder? Try *three* pails! This will be a lot harder for your dog.

TIP! Make it easier for your dog by moving the pails farther apart from each other.

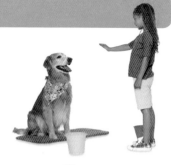

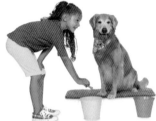

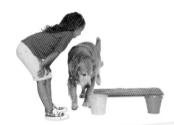

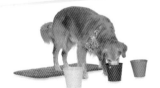

Hand Signals

Once your dog understands a hand signal, she will respond to your signal more readily than your verbal cue.

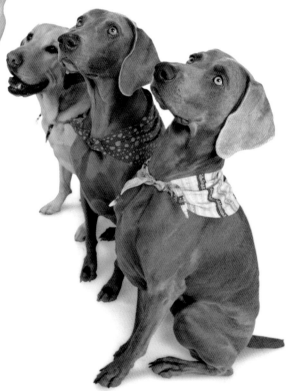

1. Hand signals are derived from the luring motion we used when initially teaching the behavior. The "sit" hand signal looks like the motion of luring the dog's head up.

2. The "down" signal appears to press the dog downward.

3. "Stay" is a traffic-cop gesture.

4. "Come" is an arm swing pulling your dog in. Hold your hand and arm rigid and make your movements clean and precise.

HOW TO TEACH IT: Start with a behavior that your dog already knows. Do the hand signal, wait one second, and then say your verbal cue. Reward your dog for doing the behavior. Your dog wants her treat as quickly as possible; she will learn that your hand signal is always followed by your verbal cue and she will learn to perform the behavior already at your hand signal in order to get her treat sooner.

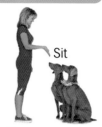
Sit

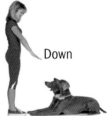
Down

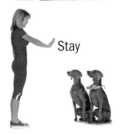
Stay

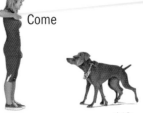
Come

Sit Pretty/Beg

This trick builds core strength, which will benefit every dog.
This trick is easier for small dogs and round dogs. Large, long,
and deep-chested dogs can may need more time to find their
balance.

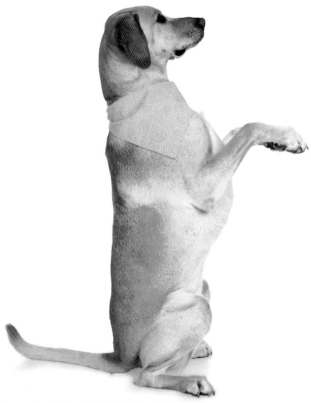

SMALL DOGS

1. Use a treat to lure your dog's head up and back. Allow him to nibble the treat, to entice him to stay in this position. If his hindquarters lift off the floor, lower your treat a little, tell him to sit, and tap his bottom down. You may wish to set your small dog on a table for easy access while training.

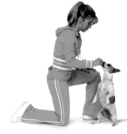

BIG DOGS

2. Position your dog in a sit. Stand directly behind him, with your heels together and your toes pointed apart.

3. Steady his chest while you lure him up. Big dogs often require several weeks or months to build the strength and coordination to hold this position on their own. The alignment of his hindquarters, thorax, forequarters, and head is key to his balance.

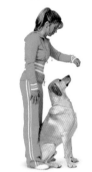

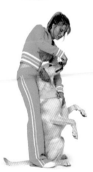

Duffle Jump

How high can you jump? Start low and work your way up.

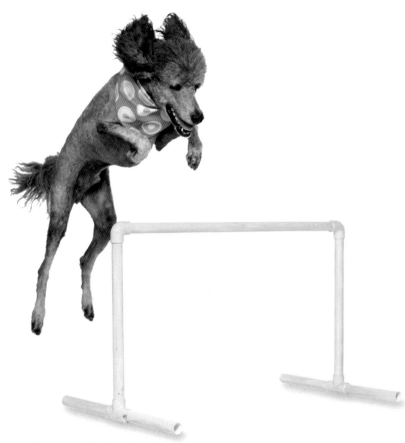

1. With your dog on a lead, jog toward a low jump and give an enthusiastic "hup!" as you jump over the bar with him. Praise him and give him a treat. If your dog is reluctant, lower the bar to the ground and walk over it with him (but don't pull him over it).

2. As your dog gains confidence, raise the jump height. Run alongside the jump now, and not over it. Make sure he has plenty of loose leash so you are not pulling his collar.

3. Can your dog go higher? Raise your arm up and over the jump to get his energy up.

TROUBLESHOOTING: If your dog tries to sneak around the side of the jump instead of over it, place the side of the jump next to a wall so he can't go around it.

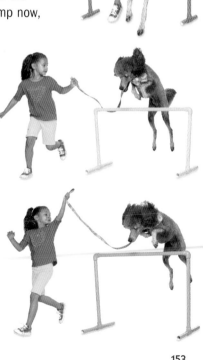

Build a Duffle Jump

SUPPLIES:

- PVC pipe (1")(2.5 cm)
- 2 PVC elbows (1")(2.5 cm)
- 2 PVC T-joints (1")(2.5 cm)
- PVC cutting tool or saw

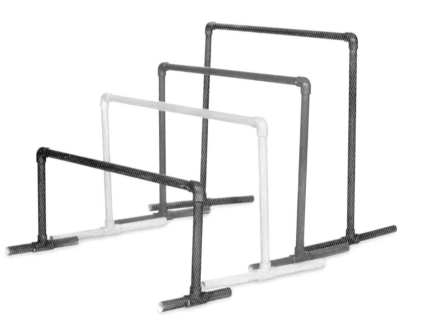

1. Cut your pipe with a PVC cutting tool or a saw. The length of the uprights will determine the height of your jump.

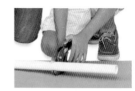

2. Assemble the two feet by pressing the pipes into the T-joints. Pound it on the ground to get a tight fit.

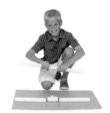

3. Assemble the two uprights.

4. Insert each upright into a foot. Lastly, insert the crossbar into the uprights.

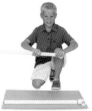

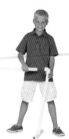

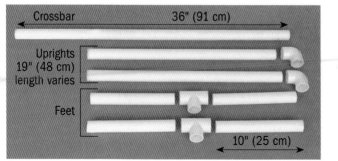

Crossbar   36" (91 cm)

Uprights 19" (48 cm) length varies

Feet

10" (25 cm)

Platform Jump

It takes courage to jump from one platform to another. Start small, and your dog will be leaping confidently in no time!

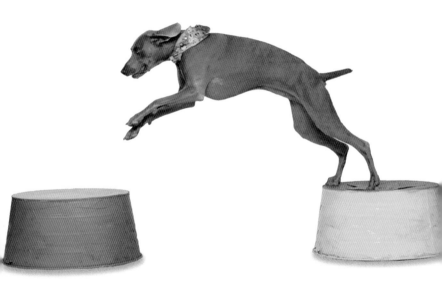

The Pocket Guide to Dog Tricks

1. Set up two adjoining platforms. Use a treat to lure your dog onto the first platform (see **paws up**, page 66). Keep moving the treat to lure her onto the second platform.

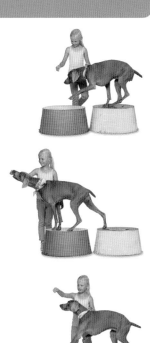

2. Give her the treat when she reaches the second platform.

3. Gradually separate the platforms so that your dog is jumping farther distances. Say "hup!" and pat the second platform. Swing your hand to give your dog the idea to jump. Always give your dog a treat on the second platform.

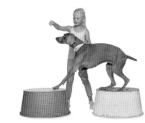

4. If your dog jumps to the ground instead of onto the second platform, place a duffle jump between the two platforms.

TIP! Platforms should be sturdy with good traction. Make sure your dog has enough landing space on the platform.

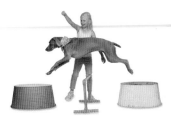

Jump Over My Back

In an impressive show of athleticism and teamwork, your dog jumps over your crouched back.

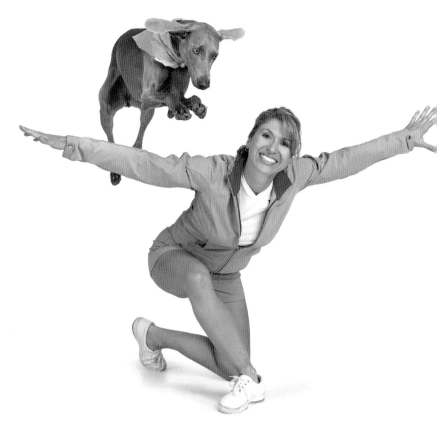

1. Stand next to the upright and have your dog **jump over a bar** (page 152). Next, kneel next to the upright as she jumps.

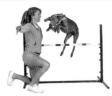

2. Kneel under the bar. Have a friend encourage your dog over if she seems reluctant.

3. Stay in position but remove the bar. Alternate jumps with the bar and without it.

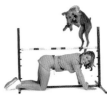

4. Lay the uprights down.

5. Remove the jump entirely. If your dog seems confused, hold the bar across your back as a visual cue.

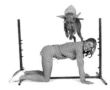

TROUBLESHOOTING: Some dogs prefer to jump on your back on their way over, while other dogs will do anything to avoid touching your back. Work with your dog to develop the method that works best for the both of you.

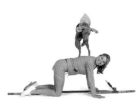

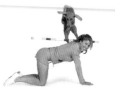

Jump Over My Knee

Kneel on the floor and have your dog jump over your knee.
Don't forget to smile!

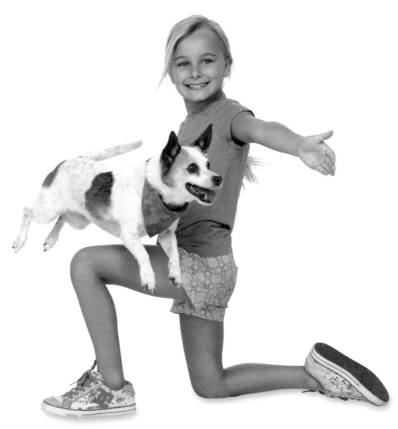

1. Sit with your legs extended and your toes against a wall. Start with your dog on your left side. Hold a treat in your right hand. Put the treat to your dog's nose so he can smell it, and move it across your legs. Hopefully, he will step or jump over your legs to get the treat.

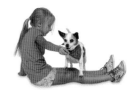

2. Kneel with your right leg outstretched, toes against the wall. Lure your dog with a treat. He may be tempted to cross near your ankle as that is the lowest spot, so hold your treat closer to your thigh. When he crosses over your leg, give him the treat.

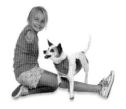

3. Raise up on your back knee and try it again.

4. Kneel with your knee against the wall. If your dog tries to go under your leg, put a cushion there to prevent him.

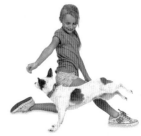

TIP! In an enthusiastic voice, say "hup!" to get a higher jump!

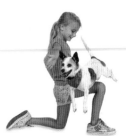

Jump into My Arms

Your dog jumps across your chest as you catch her in mid-air.

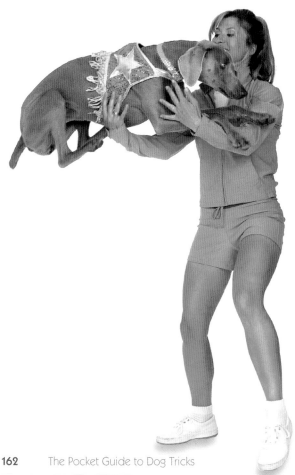

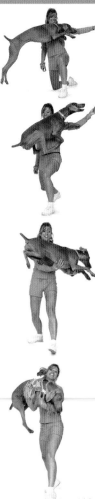

1. Have your dog **jump over your knee** (page 160). Your dog is on your left. Your right knee is raised. Hold your right hand high and away as a target for your dog.

2. Rise up slightly until your back knee is off the ground.

3. When your dog is at the apex of her jump, lightly touch her with both hands. Do not attempt a full catch the first time. Increase the pressure and duration of your grasp, concentrating on carrying her through the path of her arc and releasing her to the ground.

4. Finally, catch your dog at the highest point of her jump, continuing to swing in the direction of her travel so as not to jolt her. Avoid excessive pressure on her neck and belly.

Hoop Jump

Teach your dog to jump through a hoop like a circus dog!

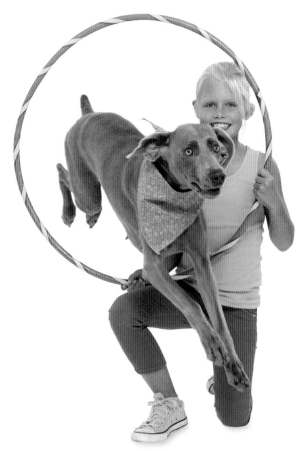

1. Remove the noisy beads from your hoop to make it less frightening for your dog. Give your dog time to investigate the hoop. Hold the hoop on the ground using the hand closest to your dog. With your other hand, use a treat to lure her through.

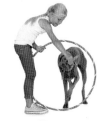

2. Raise the hoop and try again. Be prepared to drop the hoop if your dog gets tangled in it.

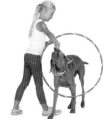

3. If your dog keeps trying to go around the hoop instead of through it, hold the hoop across a doorway.

4. Raise the hoop again so that your dog must jump to get through it. Tell her "hup!" to get her excited to jump.

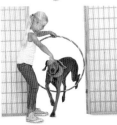

TROUBLESHOOTING: It may happen that the hoop falls on your dog and scares her. Dogs pick up on your energy, so don't make a big fuss over it. Put the hoop back down to ground level, and have her walk through it a few times.

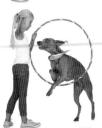

Jump through My Arms

Your dog jumps through a large circle formed by your arms.

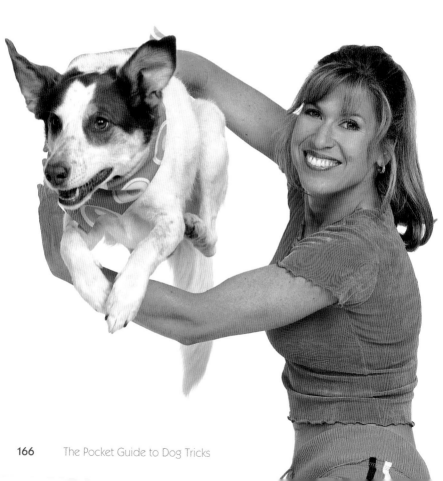

The Pocket Guide to Dog Tricks

1. Warm up with a few **hoop jumps** (page 164).

2. Gradually widen your arms around the hoop as your dog continues his jumps.

3. Set aside the hoop and cue your dog to jump through your arms only. A larger dog may require your hands to be disconnected. If your dog resists, go back to using the hoop.

4. Be creative; your dog can learn to jump through circles made with your arms or legs.

TROUBLESHOOTING: Some dogs jump easily through the hoop, but are reluctant to jump through your arms. They may be apprehensive about jumping close to your arms and head. Try alternating between the hoop and arm circles.

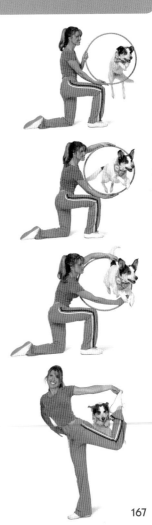

Paper-Covered Hoop

In this dramatic trick, your dog crashes through a paper-covered hoop.

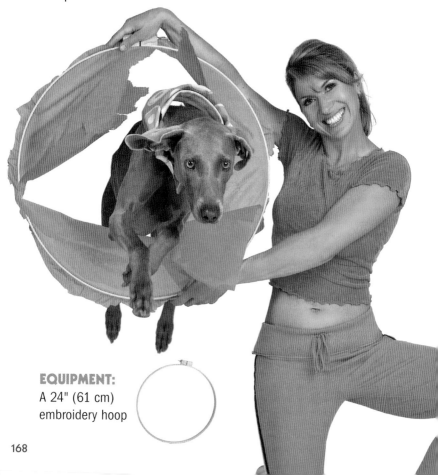

EQUIPMENT:
A 24" (61 cm) embroidery hoop

1. Practice a few **hoop jumps** (page 164), keeping the hoop low to the ground. Attach tissue paper to the top edge and lure your dog through.

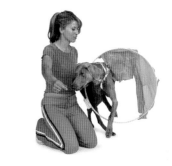

2. Cover the hoop with tissue paper, but make a big hole in the middle. Use a treat to coax your dog through the hole. It may be easier to get her to walk through rather than jump.

3. This time, just make a small hole or even just a slit. Before you know it, your dog will be comfortable breaking through the paper on her own!

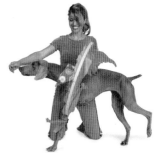

TROUBLESHOOTING: Tissue paper works best, as newspaper is pretty tough to break through without an initial slit.

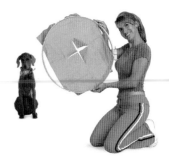

Rope Jump

You can jump rope with your dog. Use a flexible rope that is approximately 9' (2.7 m) long and 7/8" (2 cm) thick.

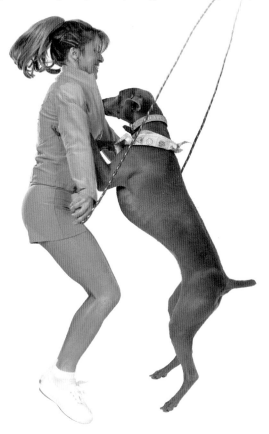

1. While your dog is in a playful mood, encourage her to jump by holding a toy or food in the air and teasing her with it. Reward even small jumps by giving her the treat or toy.

2. Next, try it without the toy. Say "hup!" and jump to encourage your dog. Hold the rope in your hand to get your dog used to it.

3. Let the rope fall lightly behind your dog and then cue her to "hup!" Reward her for jumping (even though she is not jumping over the rope at this point).

4. It will take time for your dog to learn the rhythm of the rope and the timing of your cue. Reward your dog for jumping, even if she doesn't clear the rope.

TROUBLESHOOTING: Try practicing with a hula hoop or stick. Your dog will feel it bump her ankles when she doesn't jump high enough.

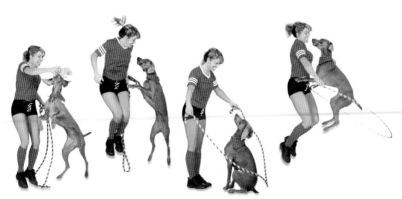

Tunnel

Going through a tunnel can be scary, at first, but with your patience and encouragement your dog will come out the other side a more confident dog.

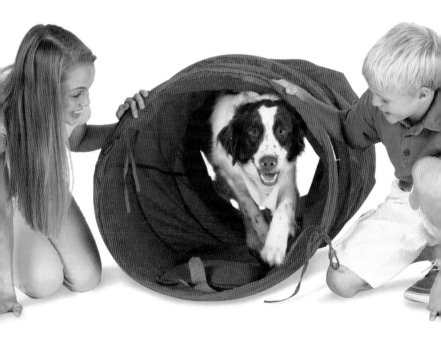

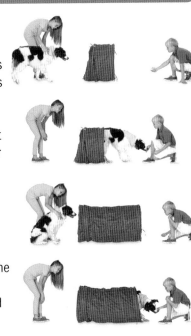

1. Collapse the tunnel and put a sand bag inside to stabilize it. One person at the tunnel entrance holds the dog, and the other person waits at the exit making eye contact with the dog through the tunnel, calling him, and holding out a treat. (Don't sit too close to the exit so that your has room to come out).

2. It may take several minutes of coaxing. When your dog finally goes through the tunnel, give him the treat.

3. Expand the tunnel. The person at the tunnel entrance must not push the dog in the tunnel but, instead, hold him until he is making eye contact with the treat, and then let him go.

4. If your dog is hesitant, put several treats inside the tunnel and let him explore it on his own. Give your dog the treat at the exit.

Commando Crawl

Teach your dog to crawl on his belly under a row of chairs, just like an army commando. This exercise builds core strength in your dog.

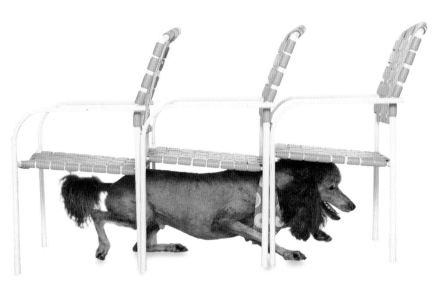

1. Put the side of a chair against a wall, so your dog can't crawl out the side. Sit on the other side of the chair so your dog can't crawl out that side, either. Use a treat to coax his head under the chair.

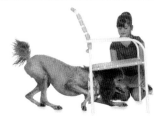

2. Tell your dog "crawl" and keep pulling the treat slowly forward. Don't move too fast, or your dog will back out.

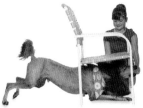

3. As your dog comes out the other side, give him the treat.

4. Now try it with two chairs. Hold treats in both of your hands, so you don't have to switch hands halfway through. Give your dog treats along the way.

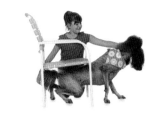

TROUBLESHOOTING: Your dog may initially try to back out of the chairs. That's okay, let him do it. Just try again, and he'll be a little more confident with every attempt.

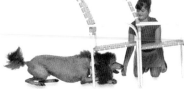

175

Ladder Work

Many dogs don't know they have back feet—their head leads them and everything else just follows. Ladder exercises teach your dog to work the mechanics of placing her feet.

EQUIPMENT:
A ladder is approximately 7 feet (2 m) long with rungs spaced 12 inches (30 cm) apart. It stands a few inches (cm) off the ground.

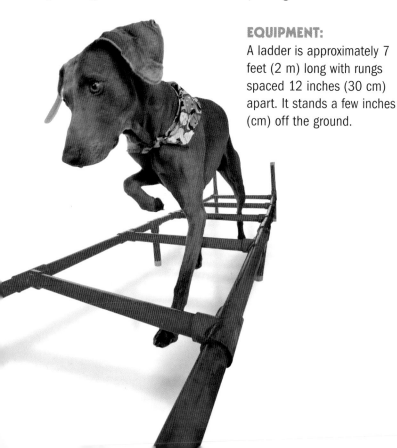

1. Place your ladder alongside a wall to prevent your dog from escaping it. Use the hand closest to your dog to hold her short leash. Hold several treats in your other hand, just above the ladder rung.

2. Lure your dog forward through two or three steps, and give her a treat (always reward low, near the rungs). Continue luring her forward with another treat.

3. Turn around and switch hands and take your dog through in the opposite direction.

4. Increase the pace as your dog gets comfortable.

TIP! Some dogs may not even like to stand still with their feet between the rungs at first. If your dog is sidestepping, squirming, or jumping, take her though the ladder more slowly.

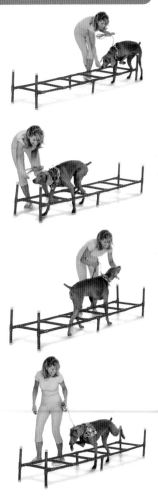

Build a Coordination Ladder

SUPPLIES

- PVC pipe (1")(2.5 cm)
  Length of approximately 22 ft (7 m)
- 4 PVC elbows (1")(2.5 cm)
- 14 PVC T-joints (1")(2.5 cm)
- PVC cutting tool or saw

CUT YOUR PVC PIPE:

8 side pieces (13" each)(33 cm)
4 half-side pieces (5.35" each)(13.5 cm)
4 spacer pieces (2" each)(5 cm)
6 rung pieces (16" each)(40 cm)
6 leg pieces (7" each)(8 cm)

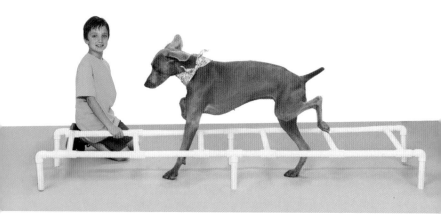

1. Cut your PVC pipe with a hand saw or a PVC cutting tool.

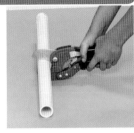

2. Lay all your pieces in place on the ground first, just like in the photo. That way you can double-check your plan.

3. Assemble the ladder boxes, working on one box at a time. Attach the elbows at the four corners. When the ladder is on the ground, the elbows should point up toward the sky.

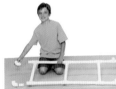

4. Insert the legs and you're done!

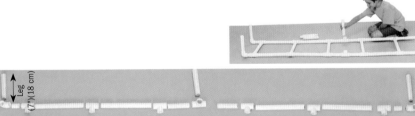

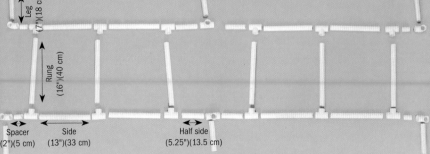

Leg (7")(18 cm)

Rung (16")(40 cm)

Spacer (2")(5 cm)

Side (13")(33 cm)

Half side (5.25")(13.5 cm)

Peekaboo

In this trick, your dog runs between your legs ... peekaboo!

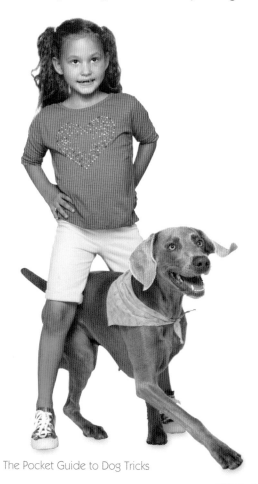

1. Turn your back to your dog. Hold a treat between your legs and wiggle it to get your dog's attention. Say, "Peekaboo!"

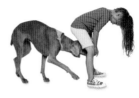

2. As your dog sniffs or nibbles at the treat, bring it slowly forward so that your dog walks between your legs. If you move too quickly, your dog will back out.

3. Once your dog is halfway through your legs, give her the treat. Let her nibble it in that position, to keep her there.

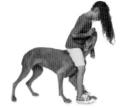

4. Over time, your dog will get braver, and will push through your legs faster.

TROUBLESHOOTING: Your dog may be scared of going between your legs. Don't hold her collar. Keep offering her treats and she'll get a little braver each time.

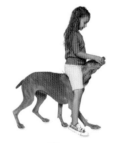

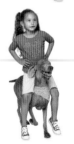

Figure-8s through My Legs

Zigzag, your dog runs in and out and between your legs making a figure-8. Now that's teamwork!

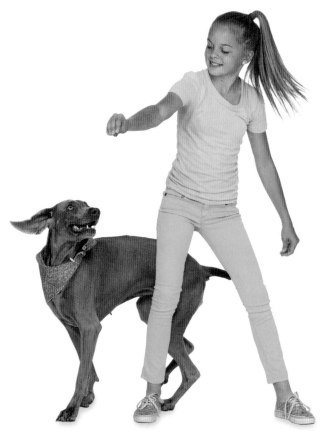

1. Hold several small treats in each hand. Your dog is at your left side. Move your left hand from her nose, forward.

2. Continue moving your left hand between your legs until your hands meet in the middle. Now get your dog to follow the treat in your right hand.

3. Give her a treat at the side of your right leg. Only reward when your dog is at the side of your leg.

4. Lure her back through your legs.

5. Have your hands meet in the middle, and your dog now follows your new hand.

6. Give her a treat by your left leg.

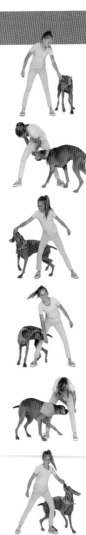

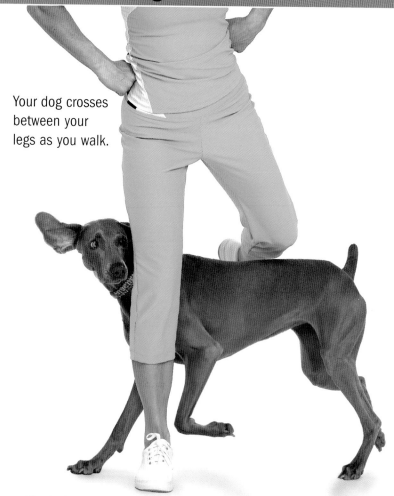

Your dog crosses between your legs as you walk.

1. Start with your dog at your left. Hold several small treats in each hand.

2. Step with your right foot. Drop your right hand straight down, between your legs. When your dog touches your hand, give her one treat. Continue to lure her all the way through your legs, giving her treats from your right hand.

3. Once she is all the way through, step with your left foot and drop your left hand straight down. Lure your dog through and give her a treat from your left hand. Repeat the steps.

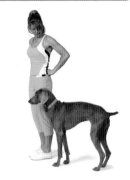

TIP! Instead of treats, you can use a short tab leash to guide your dog. Step with your right foot and pull the leash between your legs with your right hand.

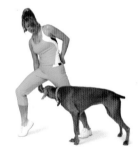

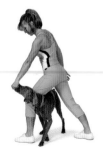

Weave poles are an obstacle in the sport of dog agility. The first pole is always passed along your dog's left shoulder, and the second pole along her right.

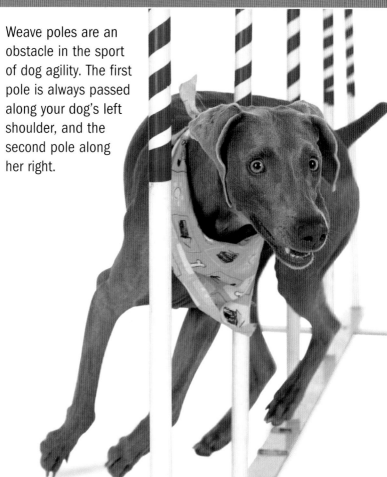

1. Start with only two poles (poles can be pointed PVC poles stuck in the grass). With your dog on your left, lead her between the poles. You can either lure her through with a treat or lead her through with a short leash.

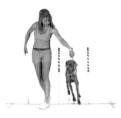

2. Stand with your dog on your left and the poles to the left of her. Lead her between the first two poles and reward her.

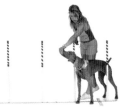

3. Have your dog weave through a series of poles.

4. Begin with your dog a few feet (60 cm) behind and to the left of the first pole. Walk forward and guide her in and out of the poles with body language by using your hand to "press" her away from you... and "pull" her back toward you.

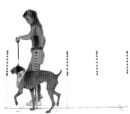

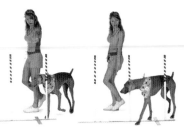

Teach "fetch" the easy way; with a squeezable hidden-treat ball. Your dog will learn to bring the ball back to you in order to get the treat.

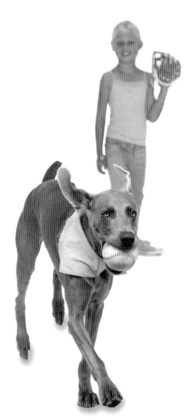

1. Use a box cutter to cut a slit in a ball.

2. Squeeze the ball to reveal the opening. Show your dog as you drop a treat inside the ball.

3. Get your dog interested in the ball by batting it around. Then playfully toss it away from her.

4. Encourage her back to you by calling and patting your legs. When you finally get the ball back, squeeze it open to let the treat drop out. Your dog will soon learn that the only way to get the treat out is to bring the ball back to you.

TROUBLESHOOTING: Never chase your dog when she is playing keep-away. Instead, lure her back with a treat or run away from her to encourage her to chase you. Have a second ball, and pretend to be having lots of fun with the new ball.

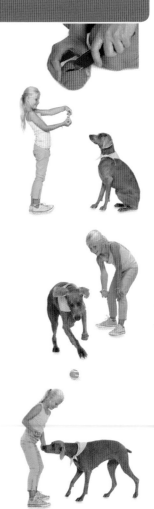

Flying Disc

Your dog will be flying high when you teach her to catch a disc! Use discs specifically designed for a dog, as toy discs are too hard for a dog's teeth.

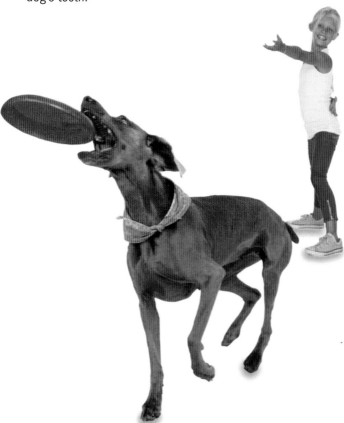

1. Spin an upside-down disc with your finger to get your dog's interest.

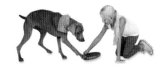

2. When she seems interested, throw a "roller" by rolling the disc along its edge. Encourage your dog to "Get it! Get it!"

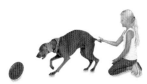

3. Pat your knees and call your dog to, "bring it back."

4. Trade her a treat for the disc.

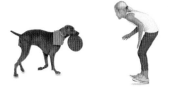

5. Throw the disc away from your dog, and not at her. If she just watches it drop, go back to rollers for a while.

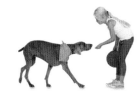

WHAT TO EXPECT: If at any point your dog loses interest in the disc, go back to the previous step. You may have to throw rollers for weeks before your dogs gets excited enough to catch one from the air.

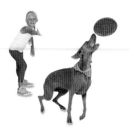

Volleyball

Toss a ball in the air and your dog will bop it back to you with her nose! This game increases coordination.

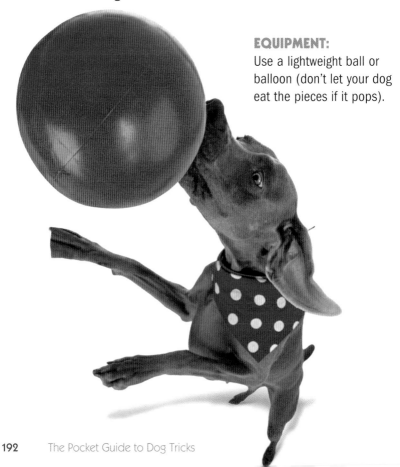

EQUIPMENT:
Use a lightweight ball or balloon (don't let your dog eat the pieces if it pops).

1. Get your dog excited to play with a plush toy. Toss it around and squeak it to get your dog's interest. Don't push it toward your dog but, rather, draw it away from her to make her chase it.

2. When your dog is focused on the toy, toss it in the air in a slow arc toward her. When she catches it, say "good!" and give her a treat.

3. While your dog is still feeling playful, switch to a lightweight ball. Toss the ball in a high arc so that it comes down rather vertically above your dog's nose.

4. Because of the large circumference of the ball, your dog will be unable to catch it, and the ball will instead bounce off her nose and back to you!

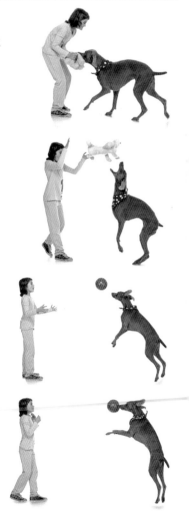

Open the Door

1. Tie some smelly treats such as steak, chicken, ham, or liver in the corner of a knotted dish towel, and wiggle it in front of your dog.

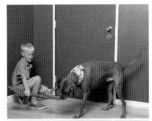

2. Tie the dish towel to the doorknob and show your dog the end with the treats. Your dog will sniff and lick the towel.

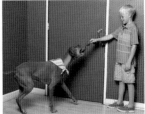

3. Encourage your dog by saying, "Get it! Open the door!" Eventually, he will pull on it a bit, and the door will move.

4. Immediately say "good!" and give him a treat from your pocket.

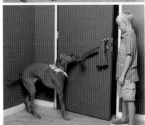

WHAT TO EXPECT: Eventually, when your dog is doing it well, take the treats out of the dish towel and instead give him a treat from your pocket when he pulls the door open.

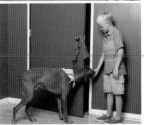

Drop It

Whether it's your shoe or a dead rat, there are times when you *really* want your dog to drop it.

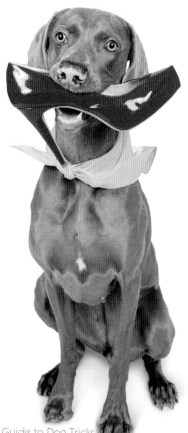

1. By using positive redirection, we will redirect your dog's attention from a bad behavior to a good behavior, and then reward that good behavior. If you were to yell "no!" your dog may run off. Instead, tell her what you *want* her to do. Show her a treat and say "drop it."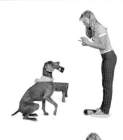

2. Keep insisting that she drop it.

3. As soon as she does, send her enthusiastically to her pedestal (page 80). You can even run with her.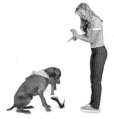

4. Reward her on the pedestal with a treat and praise. Your dog is not getting a treat for taking and then dropping the shoe; she is getting a treat for going to the pedestal. Don't worry, this will not train your dog to take more shoes! Your dog will associate the treat with the pedestal and not with the shoe. What is more likely to happen is that you'll find her spontaneously jumping on her pedestal!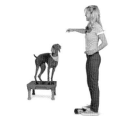

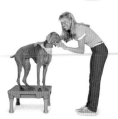

Get Your Leash

Teach your dog to fetch her leash when it's time for a walk.

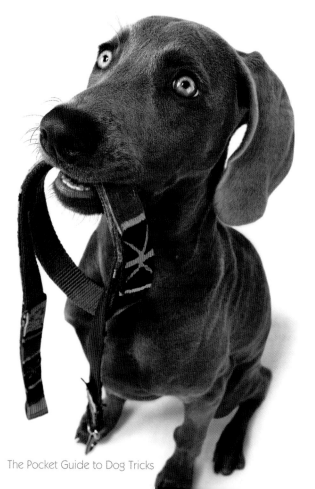

1. Teach your dog to **fetch** (page 188). Introduce the word "leash" to your dog by using it each time you put it on her. Fasten her leash together in a bundle with a rubber band and toss it playfully. Tell her to "fetch leash" and give her a treat when she returns.

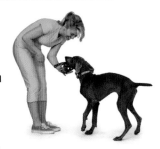

2. Now put the leash in its regular spot, such as on a table by the door. Point to it and encourage your dog to "get your leash!"

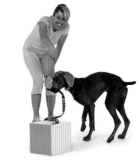

3. Reward your dog by immediately attaching her leash and taking her for a walk. Her reward now is a walk instead of a treat. The next time you are ready to go for a walk, get your dog excited to go out and then have her get her leash.

WHAT TO EXPECT: Don't be surprised if your dog communicates her wishes to you by dropping her leash in your lap! Reward her politeness as often as possible with a walk.

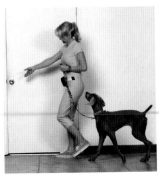

Bring Your Food Dish

Having your dog fetch his bowl before getting his dinner teaches him about working to receive rewards.

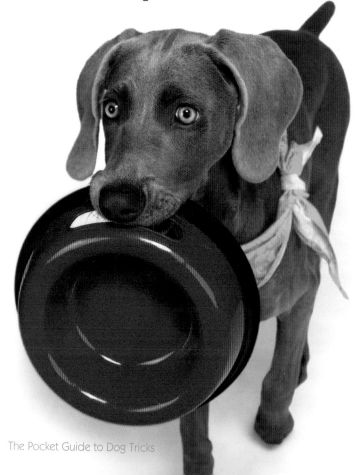

1. First, teach your dog to **fetch** (page 188). Start your routine of preparing your dog's dinner; get out the bag of dog food, etc. Point to your dog's bowl and tell her to "fetch!"

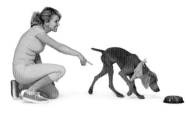

2. She will likely be excited and spinning in circles and forget what she's doing. Keep pointing to the bowl and encouraging her.

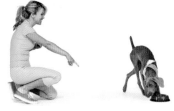

3. When she finally brings her bowl to you, praise her excitedly.

4. Immediately put her dinner or some treats in the bowl and let her eat her reward.

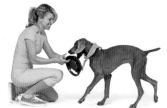

WHAT TO EXPECT: The challenge in teaching this trick will be in the first time you train it. Once your dog has one success, she will very quickly make the association between bringing her bowl and getting her dinner.

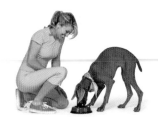

Your little helper will carry your purse or bag as you walk.

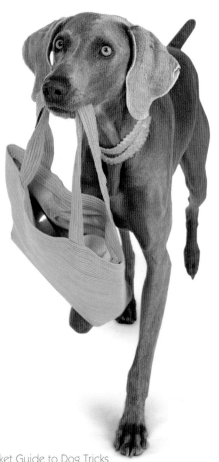

1. Put a handful of treats inside your purse and close it.

2. Hand your purse to your dog and have her take it (page 188).

3. Walk a few steps while patting your leg to indicate she should come with you. If she drops the purse, do not pick it up but rather, point to it and instruct her again to "take it."

4. Praise your dog as you take the purse and give her a treat from inside. When she realizes treats are inside the purse, she will be less likely to abandon it if she gets bored.

TROUBLESHOOTING: Dogs sometimes try to get the treats out of the purse on their own. The treats need to be inaccessible, such as in a sealed pouch.

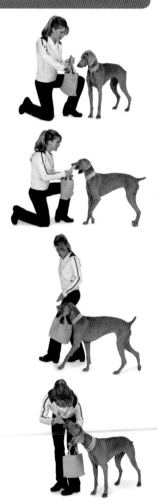

Bring Me a Tissue

Sneeze and your dog can fetch a tissue for you!

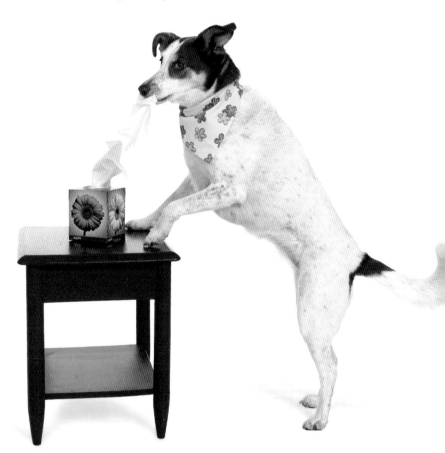

1. Secure a box of tissues to a low table or the floor using duct tape. Wiggle the tissue and tell your dog to "**take it**" (page 188). If he even puts his mouth on the tissue, say "Good!" and give him a treat. Keep practicing until he pulls the tissue out of the box.

2. Move a little away from the tissue box. Point to it and say "Achoo! Fetch!" Encourage your dog along the way, then trade him a treat for the tissue.

3. Make it harder by sneezing while sitting in a chair. If your dog drops the tissue do not pick it up, but rather encourage him to bring it the rest of the way to you.

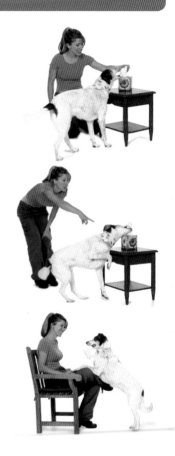

Mail from the Mailbox

Teach your dog to open the mailbox door, retrieve the mail, and close it up.

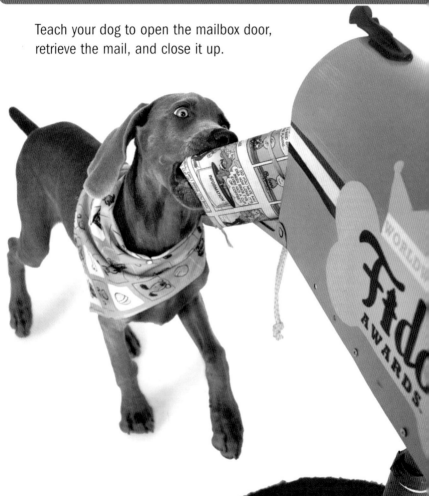

GET THE MAIL

1. Toss a rolled newspaper on the floor and have your dog to **fetch** it (page 188). Place the newspaper inside an open mailbox and have her fetch it from there.

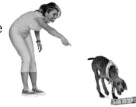

OPEN THE MAILBOX

2. Teach your dog to open the mailbox door in the same way you taught her to **open a door** (page 194).

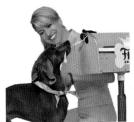

CLOSE THE MAILBOX

3. Remove the rope attached to the mailbox door, so as not to confuse your dog. Hold the door a few inches (cm) open with a string of rubber bands (the elasticity will be helpful). Dab peanut butter on the mailbox door to get your dog's interest. The moment she touches the door, say "Good!" and give her a treat.

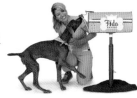

4. Next, stop rewarding for merely touching the door, and wait for her to push it closed. Once she is consistently successful, add at third rubber band to hold the door wider open and, finally, remove the rubber bands altogether.

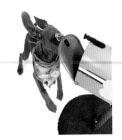

Bring Me a Beer from the Fridge

In this useful trick, your dog opens the refrigerator door, fetches a beer, and returns to close the door.

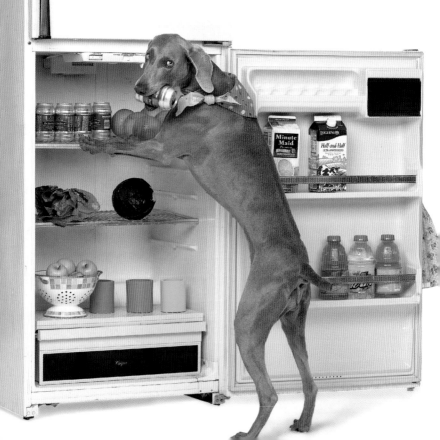

GET THE BEER

1 Play **fetch** (page 188) with an empty can to get your dog accustomed to carrying it (a foam can insulator may help). Next, place the can in an open refrigerator and have her fetch it from there.

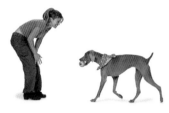

OPEN THE REFRIGERATOR

2 Teach your dog to open the refrigerator door in the same way you taught her to **open a door** (page 194). With the fridge door slightly ajar, instruct your dog to pull the dish towel. Make it more challenging by closing the fridge door completely.

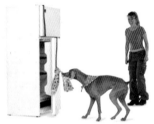

CLOSE THE REFRIGERATOR

3 Cue your dog to **close the door** (page 40) while tapping the front of the open refrigerator door. Your dog may end up using her paw to close it.

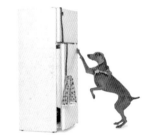

Discern Objects' Names

Your dog can learn to identify dozens of objects by name. Keep
your dog thinking by laying objects on the floor and asking her
to fetch a specific one.

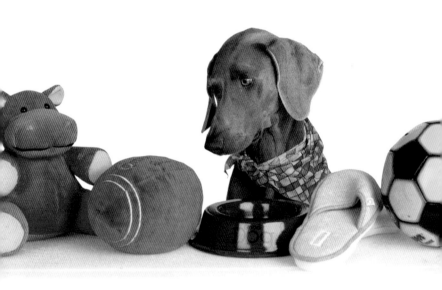

1. Start with a fun object whose name is already familiar to your dog. Lay it in a clear area alongside two other unappealing objects such as a hammer and hairbrush.

2. Point toward the objects and tell your dog to "**fetch** [toy name]" (page 188). Praise her the moment she grabs the correct object.

3. Add a second toy whose name is known to your dog. Alternate which one you tell her to find. If she chooses incorrectly, don't scold her but, rather, don't acknowledge it one way or the other. Keep telling her to "fetch [toy name]."

TROUBLESHOOTING: Your dog may be so excited that she grabs the first object she sees. Hold your dog for ten seconds as you let the words sink in. Repeat your object name several times and let her focus on the object from afar.

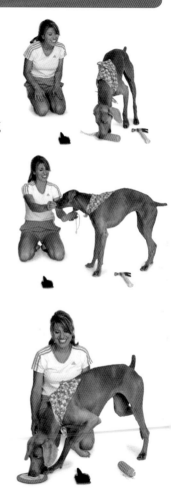

Tidy Up Toys into Toy Box

Your dog opens her toy box lid, puts her toys inside, and closes the lid.

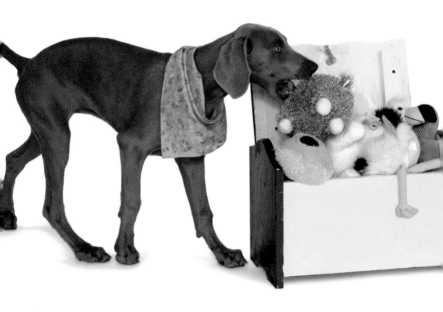

PUT AWAY THE TOY

1. Toss a toy and have your dog **fetch** (page 188). When your she returns, hold a treat slightly above the open toy box, near the lid. When she opens her mouth for the treat, the toy should fall right in. In the beginning, reward her even if the toy doesn't quite make it in.

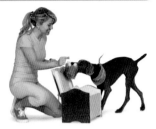

OPEN THE LID

2. Teach your dog to open the lid in the same way you taught her to **open a door** (page 194). Initially, make it easier for your dog by wedging a toy under the lid to keep it partially open.

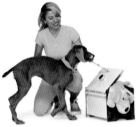

CLOSE THE LID

3. Hold the lid partially open and use a treat to lure your dog to step on the lid. When she does, allow it to fall closed and let her have the treat.

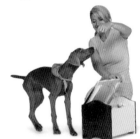

4. Gradually hold the lid farther and farther open, until your dog slams the lid without stepping on it.

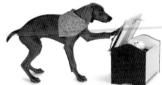

Make a Dog Toy Box

Does your dog have a lot of toys? Make her her very own box to store them in.

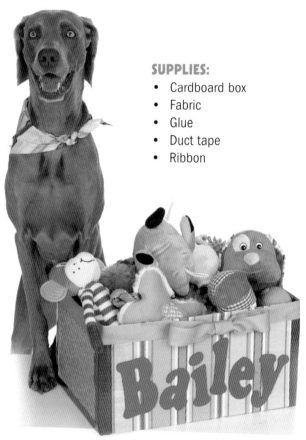

SUPPLIES:

- Cardboard box
- Fabric
- Glue
- Duct tape
- Ribbon

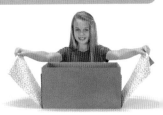

1. Start with any size cardboard box. Cut a piece of fabric the same width as the width of the box, and long enough so that it will wrap from one side of the box all the way to the other side (plus a little extra, which will fold inside the box rim). Use glue or spray adhesive to stick the fabric to the box. The ends will fold into the inside of the box.

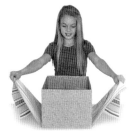

2. Cut another piece of fabric the width of the other side of your box. Again, cut it a little longer so that it wraps inside the rim of the box.

3. Glue it to the box, keeping it stretched tight. Smooth out wrinkles.

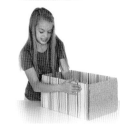

4. Use colored duct tape along each edge to cover up the seams and give it a finished look. Add a ribbon and decorations.

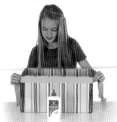

Litter in the Step Can

Teach your dog to open the step can using the foot pedal, and watch her throw the trash inside.

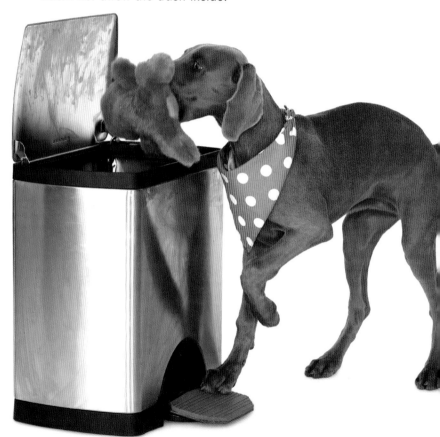

DROP THE TRASH IN THE CAN

1. Toss a toy and have your dog to **fetch** (page 188). When your dog returns hold a treat against the step can lid; when she opens her mouth for the treat, the toy should fall right in. In the beginning, give her the treat if her toy drops anywhere near the step can. You can help her by gently coax the toy in with your finger.

STEP ON THE FOOT PEDAL

2. Work on the foot pedal without the toy. If your dog knows how to **turn on a tap light** (page 74) temporarily affix the tap light onto the foot pedal to give her the idea to step on it. Otherwise, use a treat to lure your dog forward so that she accidentally steps on the pedal.

3. As she improves, your dog will learn to deliberately step on the foot pedal, and you should no longer need to lure her with a treat.

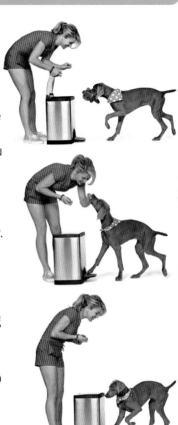

Ring Toss

Your dog maneuvers rings onto an upright pole.

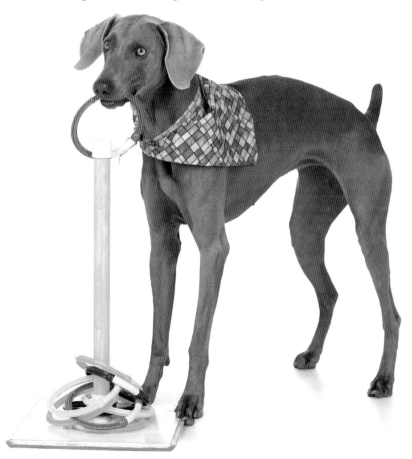

1. Have your dog to **fetch** (page 188) a ring. Hold a treat near the top of the pole to get your dog to open her mouth. When she does, use your finger to guide the ring on the pole and reward her for this.

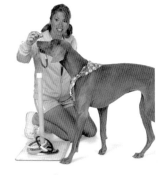

2. As your dog improves, phase out the treat and just tap the pole to focus her attention.

3. Sometimes, use your finger to guide the ring on the pole, and sometimes don't give her this help. If the ring misses the pole, say "whoops!" and try again.

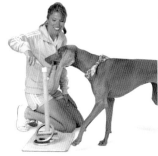

TIP! An endcap on your pole will help your dog, as she will use this to catch the bottom of the ring.

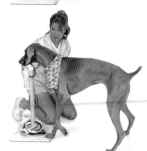

Shake Hands

Every polite pooch needs to learn to shake hands!

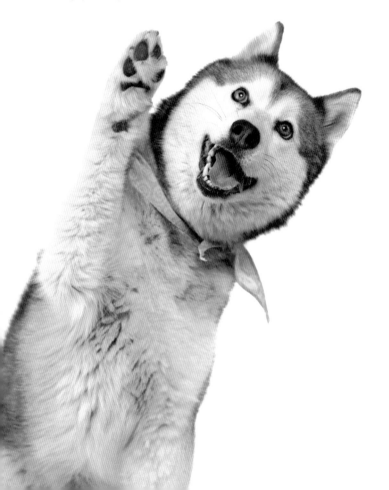

1. Hold a treat in your fist, near the ground and say "get it!" Your dog will try to poke his nose into your fist—just move your hand away a little.

2. Eventually he will get frustrated and paw at your hand—be ready for it! The instant that he lifts his paw, say "good!" and open your hand to let him have the treat. If he noses your hand at the same time that he lifts his paw, that's fine, still give him the treat. If he never lifts his paw, tap the back of his wrist to give him the idea.

3. Once your dog has the hang of this, raise your hand higher and say "shake."

4. After your dog shakes your hand, give him a treat from your other hand. It's best to give him the treat while his paw is still in your hand.

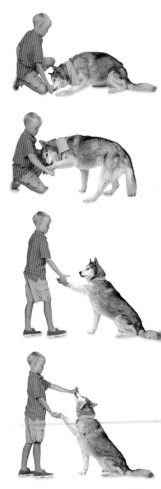

High-5

Gimme five! (Or ... actually, gimme four!)

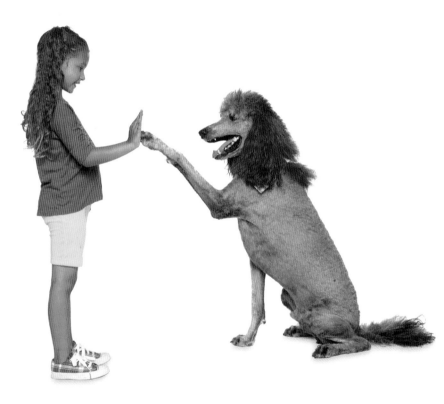

1. Have your dog **shake hands** (page 220). Give him a treat with your other hand.

2. Say "high-five, shake" and hold your hand with your fingers pointing toward the sky. Your dog won't be able to rest his paw in your hand this time, so he will probably just tap your palm. Say "good!" at the exact moment he touches your hand.

3. Give him a treat, of course.

TIP! Depending on your dog's body shape, he may not be able to reach above his shoulder. You may have to crouch down to make your hand lower.

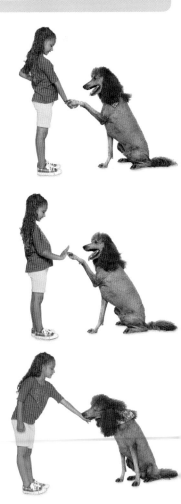

223

Pawprint Painting

Help your dog create a work of art as he spreads paint on canvas with his paws.

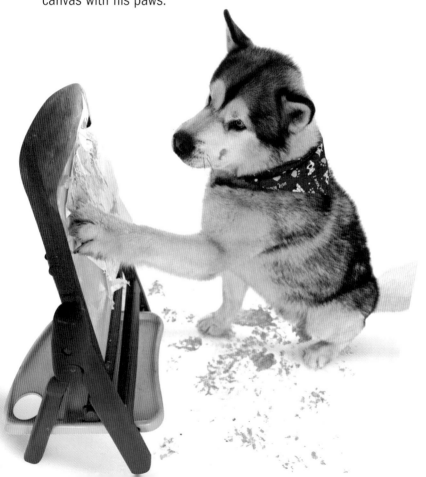

1. Have your dog **shake hands** (page 220).

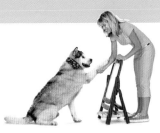

2. Next, ask your dog to "shake hands," but at the last second, pull your hand back so he is pawing at the air or at the easel. Give him a treat for this.

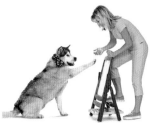

3. Pour some paint into a plate, lift your dog's paw, and press the paint onto his paw (and not his paw down into the paint).

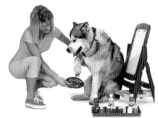

4. Stand behind the easel, hold out your hand, and ask your dog to shake hands. Again, pull your hand out of the way so he paws at the paper. Give him a treat each time that he does!

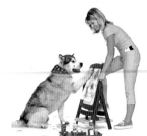

Turn Off the Light

Teach your dog to paw a light switch on the wall.

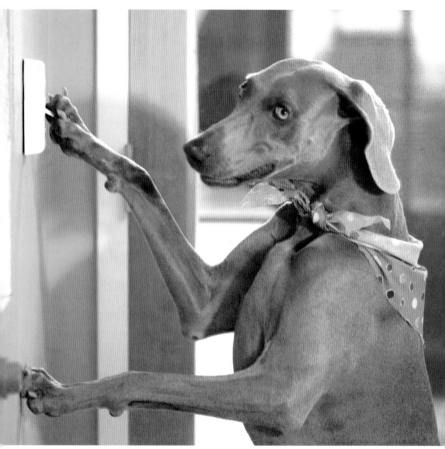

1. Hold a treat against the wall a little above the light switch and encourage your dog to "get it!" Let her have the treat when she touches the lightswitch. Hold the treat a little above the switch and away from the wall while tapping the switch with your other hand. Encourage your dog up again, but keep the treat clenched in your fist until she paws once or twice against the wall. Praise her and give her the treat while he is still upright.

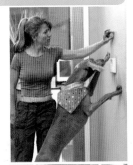

2. Tap the switch plate and say "lights!"

3. Can your dog reach the ligths on her own?

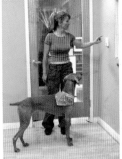

WHAT TO EXPECT: An energetic dog can pick up the concept of scratching the wall pretty quickly, however, the nuances of flipping the switch will take more time.

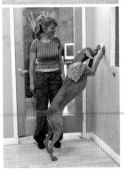

Hide Your Eyes

Your dog pretends to be shy or embarrased and cover his eyes.

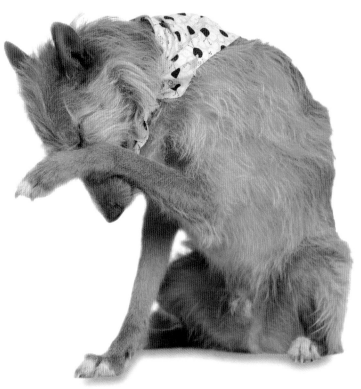

1. Stick a piece of tape on your dog's muzzle. Tap it and say "cover!"

2. Your dog will probably swat at the tape. At the exact moment that his paw touches his face, say "good!"

3. Immediately pop a treat in his mouth. (Timing is everything ... you have to react fast!)

4. After several weeks of practice, try it one time without the tape. Just tap your dog's muzzle and say "cover." If he doesn't cover his eyes, go back to using the tape for a while.

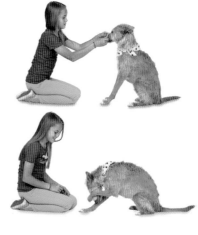

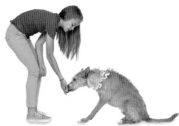

TROUBLESHOOTING: Some dogs just sit there with tape on their nose. Try sticking the tape different places: the top of his head, above or below his eye. Tap the tape a little to point it out to your dog. Encourage him by saying "get it!"

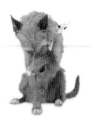

Kibble Run

Kibble rolls down the ladder of tubes and drops out the bottom for your dog.

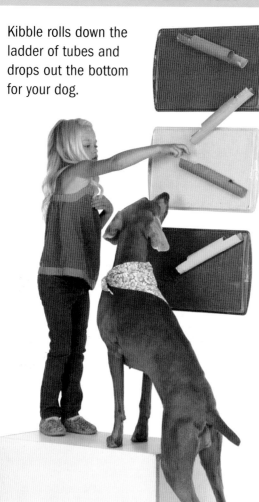

SUPPLIES

- Paper towel tubes
- Duct tape
- Small magnets
- Glue

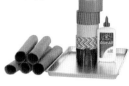

1. Cover paper towel tubes in colorful duct tape.

2. Cut off squares from both ends of the tube. These openings will catch the kibble as it falls down.

3. Glue a magnet to each end of the tube, beneath the edge of each opening that you cut.

4. Using the magnets, stick the tubes on your refrigerator or on metal cookie sheets. Arrange the tubes in a zigzag pattern.

PLAY THE KIBBLE RUN GAME:
Drop a dog food kibble in the top tube and watch it fall through all the tubes. You may have to play with it a bit until you get it just right. If the kibble makes it to the floor, your dog gets to eat it.

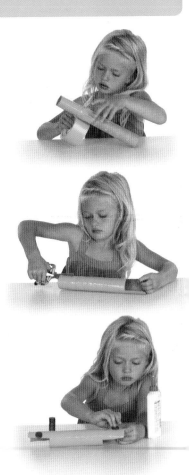

Paw Posies

In this joint art piece, your dog makes the flowers and you add the leaves and stems.

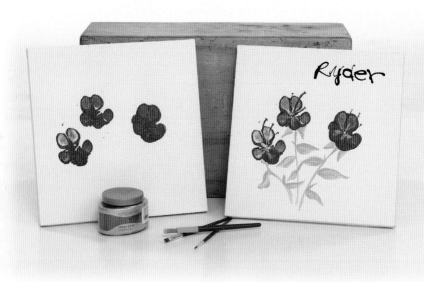

1. Pour a bright color of washable paint into a disposable plate or bowl. Tape your art paper to something sturdy like a clipboard or a cookie sheet. Set out a bowl of warm water. Lift your dog's paw by holding it just above his ankle. Lift the plate of paint up to his paw (don't try to push his paw down into the plate, as your dog will resist).

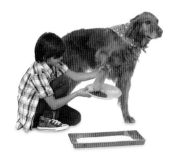

2. Lift the paper up to his paw and press for several seconds. Bring the paper straight down to avoid smudging. While the paint is drying, rinse your dog's paw in the warm water.

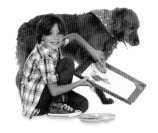

3. Pretend the paw prints are the petals of flowers and add the stems and leaves. Put a yellow dot in the center where the stigma would be.

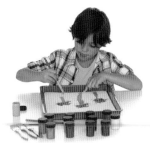

Duct Tape Treat Bag

Every dog trainer needs a treat bag. Make this stylish one in your choice of colors and patterns.

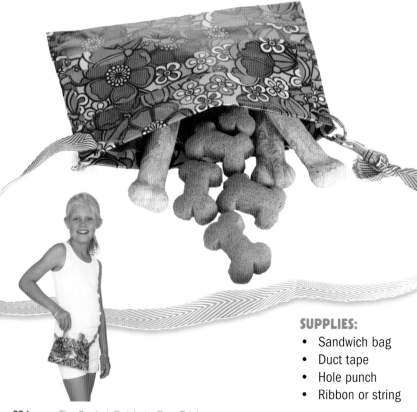

SUPPLIES:

- Sandwich bag
- Duct tape
- Hole punch
- Ribbon or string

1. Lay a zipper-seal sandwich bag on the table. Starting at the end with the opening, lay strips of duct tape across the bag. The strips should extend past the sides of the sandwich bag.

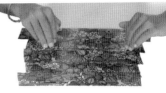

2. Flip the sandwich bag over and fold in the end pieces. Add short pieces of tape until this side is all covered.

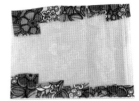

3. The bottom of the treat bag is the weakest point, so add one more piece of tape there. Fold it so it covers the bottom of the bag. Trim off the ends with scissors.

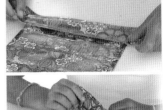

4. With scissors, cut both side seams half way.

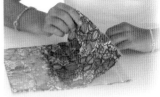

5. Fold the flaps inside the bag. Punch a hole into each of the top corners and attach a ribbon.

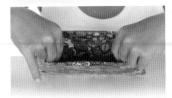

No-Mess Paw Painting

Make a masterpiece with your dog—without the mess!

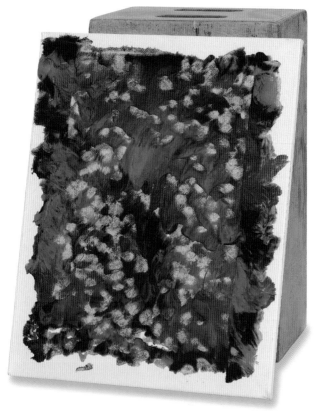

1. Choose three colors of paint. Drizzle paint onto your canvas, starting with the darkest color. You'll want to have a good amount of paint drizzled. Be sure to get all the corners.

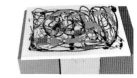

2. Lay three layers of paper towels on top of your canvas.

3. Wrap the whole thing in plastic wrap.

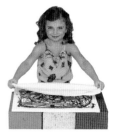

4. Hold a treat in front of your dog's nose and slowly move it away from him and toward the canvas, to get him to put his **paws up** (page 66). Have him walk across the canvas several times.

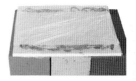

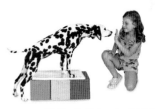

SUPPLIES

- Three colors of paint
- Canvas
- Paper towels
- Plastic wrap

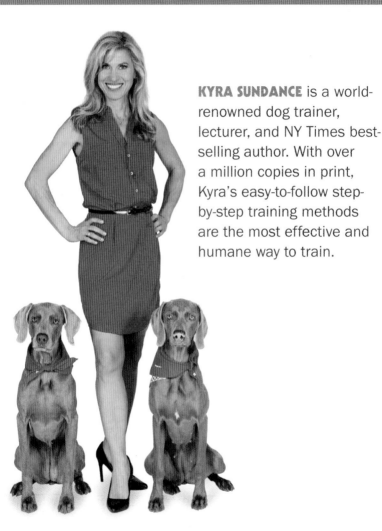

KYRA SUNDANCE is a world-renowned dog trainer, lecturer, and NY Times best-selling author. With over a million copies in print, Kyra's easy-to-follow step-by-step training methods are the most effective and humane way to train.

As professional performers, Kyra and her Weimaraners starred in shows for the king of Morocco in Marrakech, Disney's Hollywood stage shows, circuses, NBA halftime shows, on *The Tonight Show, Ellen, Animal Planet,* in movies, and in their own 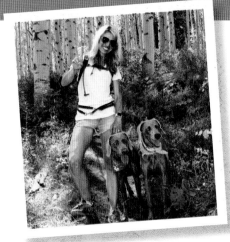 television series. Kyra is a professional set trainer for movie dogs and is nationally ranked in competitive dog sports. She presents workshops on dog tricks and canine conditioning, where her enthusiasm inspires audiences to develop fun and rewarding relationships with their own dogs.

Kyra is CEO of the *Do More With Your Dog!* trick titling organization, and chair of the *TriDEx* Trick Dog Expo.

In her spare time Kyra competes in ultramarathons.

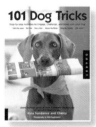
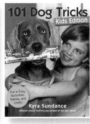
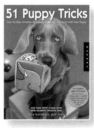
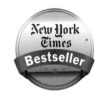
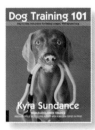
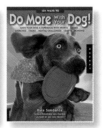
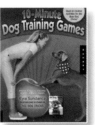
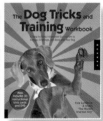
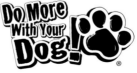